AF621004

Giuseppe Mancia
Editor

Resistant Hypertension

Epidemiology, Pathophysiology, Diagnosis and Treatment

Springer

Editor
Giuseppe Mancia
Emeritus Professor of Medicine,
University of Milano Bicocca,
IRCCS Istituto Auxologico Italiano,
Milan
Italy

ISBN 978-88-470-5570-4 ISBN 978-88-470-5415-8 (eBook)
DOI 10.1007/978-88-470-5415-8
Springer Milan Heidelberg New York Dordrecht London

Softcover re-print of the Hardcover 1st edition 2013

Printed on acid-free paper

Springer is part of Springer Science+Business Media (www.springer.com)

Resistant Hypertension

Preface

Several reasons make resistant hypertension an issue of major current interest. To mention just a few, this condition (which is defined as absence of blood pressure control despite multidrug treatment at adequate individual drug doses) is by no means rare. Although varying with the clinical setting in which resistant hypertension is studied, the consensus is that this condition may affect about 10% of the overall hypertensive population, which amounts to more than 6 million patients in the USA and more than 10 millions in Europe.

Secondly, patients with resistant hypertension have a high cardiovascular risk, with a much greater chance of developing heart failure, cerebrovascular or coronary disease, and endstage renal disease than patients in which blood pressure is more easily controlled.

Thirdly, there is a great deal of uncertainty on which antihypertensive drugs should be added when the three-drug regimen turns out to be ineffective or only partially effective. All drugs with mechanisms of action different from the currently administered ones have a chance of leading to some blood pressure reduction, but for each of them the effect involves only a limited number of cases and little information is available on: 1) whether some drugs are on average better than others and 2) which drug has a greater chance to work in which patient.

Finally, recent studies suggest that in resistant hypertension blood pressure can be reduced with invasive procedures such as renal denervation and carotid baroreceptor stimulation, pointing to sympathetic hyperactivity as an important mechanism in the maintenance of the persistent blood pressure elevation. Although the evidence is still incomplete, this represents a new promising therapeutic approach, whose availability has greatly stimulated research in this area. A demonstration is the striking, progressive increase in the number of studies on resistant hypertension which have taken place in the last 4 years, with new information not only on its treatment but also on its epidemiological, pathophysiological and diagnostic aspects.

This book has been designed to present this new information in a coordinated fashion, the aim being to offer a comprehensive view of this hot area of cardiovascular medicine. The chapters range from epidemiology to pathophysiology, diagnosis and treatment of individuals with a persistently high blood pressure, and treatment includes the potential of both antihypertensive drugs and of new invasive therapeutic approaches. All authors are experts whose research has contributed to collection of the data. I hope physicians will enjoy the reading and find it useful for their practice.

Giuseppe Mancia

Contents

Resistant Hypertension: Definition, Prevalence, and Cardiovascular Risk

1

Renata Cífková

1.1 Introduction

Hypertension is the most common cardiovascular disorder affecting 20–50% of the adult population, with a steep increase with aging [1, 2].

Elevated blood pressure (BP) has been identified as a risk factor for stroke, heart failure, coronary heart disease (CHD), peripheral arterial disease, renal failure, and, more recently, atrial fibrillation [3–6].

Data from observational studies involving 1 million individuals have indicated that death from both CHD and stroke increases progressively and linearly from BP levels as low as 115 mmHg systolic and 75 mmHg diastolic [7]. The increased risks are present in all age groups ranging from 40 to 89 years old. For every 20 mmHg systolic or 10 mmHg diastolic increase in BP, there is a doubling of mortality from both CHD and stroke.

Hypertension is poorly controlled worldwide. Epidemiological studies in various European and non-European countries show that no more than one-quarter or, at best, one-third of treated hypertensive patients achieve BP values <140/90 mmHg. The rates of hypertension treatment and control in Europe are lower than in the USA or Canada [8], a fact supported by lower stroke mortality rates in

R. Cífková (✉)
Center for Cardiovascular Prevention, Charles University in Prague,
First Faculty of Medicine and Thomayer Hospital,
Videnska 800, 140 59, Prague 4, Czech Republic

Department of Medicine II, Charles University Medical School I, Prague, Czech Republic

International Clinical Research Center, St. Anne's University Hospital Brno,
Brno, Czech Republic
e-mail: renata.cifkova@ftn.cz

G. Mancia (ed.), *Resistant Hypertension*, DOI: 10.1007/978-88-470-5415-8_1,

the two North American countries. Suboptimal BP control is consequently the most common attributable risk for death worldwide [9].

Several large hypertension outcome trials also demonstrated a failure to achieve BP goals in spite of protocol-defined treatment regimens. In these trials, 20–35% of participants could not achieve BP control despite receiving >3 antihypertensive medications [10–12].

1.2 Definitions of Resistant Hypertension

There is no uniform definition of resistant hypertension (Table 1.1).

The 2003 European Society of Hypertension-European Society of Cardiology guidelines for the management of arterial hypertension were the first to use the term resistant hypertension when a therapeutic plan that has included attention to lifestyle measures and the prescription of at least three drugs at adequate doses has failed to lower systolic and diastolic BP sufficiently [13]. The 2007 guidelines for the management of arterial hypertension, again developed jointly by the same two European societies, used virtually the same definition of resistant hypertension, with the addition of a diuretic as one of the three drugs [14].

Later in the same year, resistant hypertension was defined by the Seventh Report of the US Joint National Committee on Prevention, Detection, Evaluation and Treatment of High BP (JNC 7) as a failure to achieve goal BP < 140/90 mmHg [or <130/80 mmHg in patients with diabetes or chronic kidney disease (CKD)] in patients with hypertension who are adherent to maximal tolerated doses of an appropriate regimen consisting of three antihypertensive drugs, one of which is a diuretic [15]. This definition is not applicable to recently diagnosed

Table 1.1 The most frequently used definitions of resistant hypertension

2003 ESH-ESC guidelines
Failure of a therapeutic plan that has included attention to lifestyle measures and the prescription of at least three drugs at adequate doses to lower systolic and diastolic blood pressure sufficiently
2007 ESH-ESC guidelines
Failure of a therapeutic plan that has included attention to lifestyle measures and the prescription of at least three drugs (including a diuretic) at adequate doses to lower systolic and diastolic blood pressure to goal
JNC 7 (2003)
Failure to achieve goal blood pressure (<140/90 or <130/80 mmHg in patients with diabetes or CKD) in patients who are adhering to full doses of an appropriate three-drug regimen that includes a diuretic
AHA 2008
Blood pressure that remains above goal in spite of the concurrent use of three antihypertensive agents of different classes; ideally, one of the three agents should be a diuretic, and all agents should be prescribed at optimal dose amounts

hypertensive patients and/or those who have not yet been treated regardless of their BP levels [16]. The same definition was adopted by the American Heart Association (AHA) in its position statement on resistant hypertension [17]. The AHA position statement suggests that this definition—while arbitrary regarding the number of failed medications required—provides clarity for the clinician in that it identifies high-risk patients with curable (secondary) causes of hypertension as well as patients who, because of persistently high BP levels, may benefit from specific diagnostic testing. By this definition, resistant hypertension includes patients whose BP is controlled with the use of more than three medications, that is, patients whose BP is controlled using four or more medications. The AHA scientific statement describes these patients as having controlled resistant hypertension (Table 1.2).

There has been ongoing discussion whether the definition of resistant hypertension should include treatment with mineralocorticoid receptor antagonists, suggested as step 4 for treatment of resistant hypertension by the 2011 NICE Guideline [18].

Many patients who present as having resistant hypertension actually do not have it; this condition is called pseudoresistant hypertension. Several factors may produce the perception of resistant hypertension (Table 1.3). Thus, physicians

Table 1.2 Definitions of various forms of resistant hypertension

Resistant hypertension
Failure to achieve goal blood pressure (<140/90 mmHg) using a minimum of three antihypertensive drugs at maximal tolerated doses, one of which must be a diuretic
Controlled resistant hypertension
Patients who meet the definition of resistant hypertension but whose blood pressure is controlled at maximal tolerated doses of four or more antihypertensive medications
Refractory hypertension
Patient who meet the definition of resistant hypertension but whose blood pressure is not controlled on maximal tolerated doses of four or more antihypertensive medications
Pseudoresistant hypertension
Apparent lack of BP control under appropriate treatment in a patient who does not actually have resistant hypertension

Table 1.3 Factors related to pseudoresistant hypertension

• Improper blood pressure measurement technique
• Heavily calcified or atherosclerotic arteries difficult to compress
• Poor patient adherence to lifestyle measures and antihypertensive medication
• White-coat effect
• Suboptimal drug treatment of hypertension (improper combination, absence of a diuretic, inadequate doses)

should carefully evaluate the patient to exclude such factors before labeling someone as resistant hypertensive, and perform further diagnostic tests.

1.3 Prevalence of Resistant Hypertension

So far, the prevalence of resistant hypertension has not been properly examined. A more accurate determination would ideally be possible with prospective cohort studies coming from the general population including large subgroups of patients with hypertension. A mandatory increase in medication dosage to achieve goal BP and ensured adherence to treatment with maximal tolerated doses of at three antihypertensive medications including a diuretic should be part of the study protocol.

1.3.1 Specialized Centers

The prevalence of resistant hypertension was first examined in retrospective studies of selected populations from tertiary referral centers. A report from the Yale University Hypertension Center, Connecticut, USA, covering the 1986–1988 period included 436 patients referred for hypertension; 91 of them (20.9%) met the criteria for resistant hypertension [19]. In the majority of these patients, BP control was achieved or BP significantly improved. Only few patients had true resistant hypertension, and most of them had pseudoresistant hypertension (suboptimal medical regimen, medical intolerance, previous undiagnosed secondary hypertension, non-compliance, psychiatric causes, and drug interaction).

Another cohort of 1,281 patients referred to the RUSH University Hypertension Center, Chicago, Illinois, USA, for uncontrolled hypertension between 1993 and 2001 showed an 11% prevalence of resistant hypertension. Of these, 94% had uncontrolled hypertension for various reasons [20].

A retrospective analysis of referrals to the tertiary hypertension clinic at the University of Alabama at Birmingham, USA, over an 8-year period provided further evidence that BP could be controlled in patients referred for hypertension. Actually, only 29 of 304 patients (9.5%) referred for resistant hypertension remained refractory to treatment after careful evaluation and appropriate management including at least three visits to a hypertension clinic with a minimum follow-up of 6 months [21].

In a Spanish Ambulatory Blood Pressure Monitoring (ABPM) Registry, a total of 8,295 patients were found to have office BP $\geq$ 140 and/or 90 mmHg while treated with $\geq$3 antihypertensive agents at appropriate doses, resulting in a prevalence of 12.2% in the treated hypertensive population [22]. The Spanish ABPM Registry is a unique database coming from primary care centers and specialized units across the country and having information on more than 68,000 treated hypertensive patients.

The prevalence of resistant hypertension seems to be particularly high in nephrology clinics [23], where it may exceed 50% depending largely on the stage of the underlying CKD that led to the referral [24].

1.3.2 Subgroup Analysis of Large Clinical Trials

Extrapolation of data from large clinical trials should be done with caution because medication is provided for free, adherence is closely monitored, and titration of therapy is guided by the study protocol. In addition to that, resistant hypertension was an exclusion criterion for most studies. A combination of three drugs from different classes was not always feasible in these studies because the protocol was designed to test agents from a specific drug class. As diuretics were not allowed in some of the studies, the patients actually did not meet the criteria for resistant hypertension.

This is exemplified by the Antihypertensive and Lipid-Lowering Treatment to Prevent Heart Attack Trial (ALLHAT) where 27.3% of patients were taking three or more antihypertensive drugs at study completion after 8 years, but only 66% of patients had achieved their goal BP (68% of patients in the chlorthalidone, 66.3% in the amlodipine, and 61.2% in the lisinopril groups). Thus, the prevalence of resistant hypertension, with all the above limitations, was 17.2% [25].

1.3.3 Epidemiological Studies

A retrospective observational study, reviewing electronic medical records, was conducted in an approx. 100 US practice sites involving 2,700, mostly primary care, physicians. A diagnosis of resistant hypertension based on the AHA criteria was 9.1% of the 29,474 adult patients diagnosed with hypertension who had attended annual follow-up visits [26].

Persell used the NHANES data from 2003 to 2008 with the aim to provide a population-based estimate of the prevalence of resistant hypertension in the USA. In this study, resistant hypertension was defined as a BP $\geq$ 140/90 mmHg in patients who reported use of antihypertensive medications from three different drug classes in the past month, or who reported use of antihypertensive medications from four or more drug classes in the past month regardless their BP levels [27]. This represented 12.8% of the antihypertensive drug-treated population. Most of these individuals (85.6%) used a diuretic. Cardiovascular disease, diabetes, obesity, and renal dysfunction were common in this population of resistant hypertension.

In a subsequent study [28] published in 2011, three NHANES data sets (1988–1994, 1999–2004, and 2005–2008) were used to estimate trends in the prevalence of resistant hypertension during 1988 and 2008. In this study, uncontrolled hypertension was defined as BP $\geq$ 140/90 mmHg and apparent treatment-resistant hypertension was defined as BP ≥ 140/90 mmHg despite reported use of at least three antihypertensive medications. Within the period of 1988 and 2008, the proportion of patients with uncontrolled hypertension declined from 73.2 to 52.5%. However, the prevalence of apparent treatment-resistant hypertension (calculated as a proportion of the treated hypertensive population) increased significantly from 15.9 to 28.0%. Clinical characteristics of patients with apparent treatment-resistant hypertension included obesity, CKD, and Framingham 10-year coronary risk >20%.

1.4 Cardiovascular Risk

Cardiovascular risk and prognosis of patients with resistant hypertension compared with those having more easily controlled hypertension have not been specifically evaluated. Such patients typically present with a long-standing history of poorly controlled hypertension and commonly have associated cardiovascular risk factors such as diabetes, obstructive sleep apnea, and/or CKD. While their prognosis is likely to be unfavorable, the benefits of successful treatment may be substantial (as suggested by Veteran Administration Cooperative Studies).

Quite recent studies suggest that ABPM may have a special role in assessing cardiovascular risk in resistant hypertension. A prospective cohort study of 556 resistant hypertensive patients showed that higher ambulatory BP predict cardiovascular morbidity and mortality in resistant hypertension whereas office BP has no prognostic value [29]. Subsequent analyses by the same authors showed that other parameters derived from ABPM recordings such as non-dipping nighttime BP pattern and ambulatory arterial stiffness thickness were also independently associated with cardiovascular morbidity and mortality [30, 31].

Previous case–control studies showed that patients with resistant hypertension carry a higher burden of target organ damage (such as left ventricular hypertrophy, carotid intima-media thickening, retinal lesions, and microalbuminuria) than those with satisfactory BP control [32]. There is also some evidence that true resistant hypertension is associated with high urinary albumin excretion [33]. The Spanish ABPM Registry found that a nighttime systolic BP is more closely associated with high urinary albumin excretion rates than any other ABPM parameter in patients with resistant hypertension.

Whether the cardiovascular risk related to resistant hypertension is reduced with adequate therapy has not been evaluated. The benefits of successful treatment in these individuals are likely to be substantial; this could only be extrapolated from major outcome studies where the greater the baseline BP levels and/or the larger the decrease in BP, the greater the reductions in hypertension-associated target organ damage [34].

Acknowledgments Development of this chapter was supported by the European Regional Development Foundation—Project FNUSA-ICRC (No. CZ.1.05/1.1.00/02.0123).

References

1. Kearney PM, Whelton M, Reynolds K et al (2004) Worldwide prevalence of hypertension: a systematic review. J Hypertens 22:11–19
2. Pereira M, Lunet N, Azevedo A et al (2009) Differences in prevalence, awareness, treatment control of hypertension between developing and developed countries. J Hypertens 27:963–975
3. MacMahon S, Peto R, Cutler J et al (1990) Blood pressure, stroke, and coronary heart disease. Part 1, Prolonged differences in blood pressure: prospective observational studies corrected for the regression dilution bias. Lancet 335:765–774
4. Kannel WB (1996) Blood pressure as a cardiovascular risk factor: prevention and treatment. JAMA 275:1571–1576
5. Walker WG, Neaton JD, Cutler JA et al (1992) Renal function change in hypertensive members of the Multiple risk factor intervention trial: racial and treatment effects. The MRFIT Research Group. JAMA 268:3085–3091
6. Benjamin EJ, Levy D, Vaziri SM et al (1994) Independent risk factors for atrial fibrillation in a population-based cohort: the Framingham Heart Study. JAMA 271:840–844
7. Lewington S, Clarke R, Qizilbash N et al (2002) Age-specific relevance of usual blood pressure to vascular mortality: a meta-analysis of individual data for one million adults in 61 prospective studies. Prospective studies collaboration. Lancet 360:1903–1913
8. Wolf-Maier K, Cooper RS, Banegas JR et al (2003) Hypertension prevalence and blood pressure levels in 6 European countries, Canada and the United States. JAMA 289:2363–2369
9. World Health Report (2002) Reducing risks, promoting healthy life. World Health Organization, Geneva
10. ALLHAT Officers and Coordinators for the ALLHAT Collaborative Research Group. The Antihypertensive and Lipid-Lowering Treatment to Prevent Heart Attack Trial (2002) Major outcomes in high-risk hypertensive patients randomized to angiotensin-converting enzyme inhibitor or calcium channel blocker vs diuretic: ALLHAT. JAMA 288:2981–2997
11. Dahlof B, Devereux RB, Kjeldsen SE et al (2002) Cardiovascular morbidity and mortality in the Losartan Intervention for Endpoint reduction in hypertension study (LIFE): a randomised trial against atenolol. Lancet 359:995–1003
12. Pepine CJ, Handberg EM, Cooper-DeHoff RM et al (2003) A calcium antagonist vs a non-calcium antagonist hypertension treatment strategy for patients with coronary artery disease. The International Verapamil-Trandolapril Study (INVEST): a randomized controlled trial. JAMA 290:2805–2816
13. European Society of Hypertension-European Society of Cardiology Guidelines Committee (2003) 2003 European society of hypertension–European society of cardiology guidelines for the management of arterial hypertension. Guidelines committee. J Hypertens 21:1011–1053
14. Mancia G, De Backer G, Dominiczak A et al (2007) 2007 Guidelines for the management of arterial hypertension: the task force for the management of arterial hypertension of the European society of hypertension (ESH) and of the European society of cardiology (ESC). J Hypertens 25:1105–1187
15. Chobanian AV, Bakris GL, Black HR et al (2003) Seventh report of the joint national committee on prevention, detection, evaluation, and treatment of high blood pressure. Hypertens 42:1206–1252
16. Moser M, Setaro JF (2006) Clinical practice. Resistant or difficult-to-control hypertension. N Engl J Med 355:385–392
17. Calhoun DA, Jones D, Textor S et al (2008) Resistant hypertension: diagnosis, evaluation, and treatment: a scientific statement from the American heart association professional education committee of the council for high blood pressure research. Circulation 117: e510–e526
18. http://guidance.nice.org.uk/CG127/Guidance/pdf/English

19. Yakovlevitch M, Black HR (1991) Resistant hypertension in a tertiary care clinic. Arch Int Med 151:1786–1792
20. Garg JP, Elliott WJ, Folker A et al (2005) Resistant hypertension revisited: a comparison of two university-based cohorts. Am J Hypertens 18:619–626
21. Acelajado MC, Pisoni R, Dudenbostel T et al (2012) Refractory hypertension: definition, prevalence, and patient characteristics. Clin Hypertens 14:7–12 (Greenwich)
22. De Nicola L, Borrelli S, Gabbai FB et al (2011) Burden of resistant hypertension in hypertensive patients with non-dialysis chronic kidney disease. Kidney Blood Press Res 34:58–67
23. Kaplan NM (2005) Resistant hypertension. J Hypertens 23:1441–1444
24. ALLHAT Officers and Coordinators for the ALLHAT Collaborative Research Group (2005) The antihypertensive and lipid-lowering treatment to prevent heart attack trial. Major outcomes in moderately hypercholesterolemic, hypertensive patients randomized to pravastatin vs usual care: the antihypertensive and lipid-lowering treatment to prevent heart attack trial (ALLHAT-LLT). JAMA 288:2998–3007
25. McAdam-Marx C, Ye X, Sung JC et al (2009) Results of a retrospective, observational pilot study using electronic medical records to assess the prevalence and characteristics of patients with resistant hypertension in an ambulatory care setting. Clin Ther 31:1116–1123
26. Persell SD (2011) Prevalence of resistant hypertension in the United States, 2003–2008. Hypertension 57:1076–1080
27. de la Sierra A, Segura J, Banegas JR et al (2011) Clinical features of 8295 patients with resistant hypertension classified on the basis of ambulatory blood pressure monitoring. Hypertension 57:898–902
28. Egan BM, Zhao Y, Axon RN et al (2011) Uncontrolled and apparent treatment resistant hypertension in the United States, 1988–2008. Circulation 124:1046–1058
29. Salles GF, Cardoso CR, Muxfeldt ES (2008) Prognostic influence of office and ambulatory blood pressures in resistant hypertension. Arch Int Med 168:2340–2346
30. Muxfeldt ES, Cardoso CR, Salles GF (2009) Prognostic value of nocturnal blood pressure reduction in resistant hypertension. Arch Int Med 169:874–880
31. Muxfeldt ES, Cardoso CR, Dias VB et al (2010) Prognostic impact of the ambulatory arterial stiffness index in resistant hypertension. J Hypertens 28:1547–1553
32. Cuspidi C, Macca G, Sampieri L et al (2001) High prevalence of cardiac and extracardiac target organ damage in refractory hypertension. J Hypertens 19:2063–2070
33. Oliveras A, Armario P, Hernández-Del Rey R et al (2010) Urinary albumin excretion is associated with true resistant hypertension. J Hum Hypertens 24:27–33
34. Collins R, Peto R, MacMahon S, Hebert P et al (1990) Blood pressure, stroke, and coronary heart disease. Part 2, short-term reductions in blood pressure: overview of randomised drug trials in their epidemiological context. Lancet 335:827–838

Part I
Pathophysiology

Resistant Hypertension: Neurohumoral Aspects

2

Gian Paolo Rossi

2.1 Introduction

Even though more than one hundred antihypertensive drugs are available, alone or in combination, to fight high blood pressure (BP), the rate of control of arterial hypertension remains far from optimal worldwide. In a substantial proportion of the patients referred to specialized hypertension clinics for drug-resistant hypertension (RH), high BP is only one of the signs of underlying diseases (enlisted in Table 2.1), which are associated with neurohumoral mechanisms. Thus, the purpose of this chapter is to review these conditions and the role of activation of these mechanisms.

2.2 Renin–Angiotensin–Aldosterone System

Renovascular hypertension (RVH) can be a common cause of RH: When obstruction of one or both renal arteries narrows the vessel lumen by more than 75 % (but even less severe narrowing indicates heamodynamically relevant stenosis if there is post-stenotic dilatation), the decrease in renal perfusion pressure triggers renin secretion, thus raising BP. As RVH is potentially reversible, it should be timely identified not only to resolve RH, but also because if unrecognized, RVH can lead to end-stage kidney disease and prominent cardiovascular (CV) disease.

There is no conflict of interest and no financial disclosure concerning this chapter to be disclosed.

G. P. Rossi (✉)
Department of Medicine—DIMED, Clinica Medica 4, University Hospital,
Via Giustiniani 2, 31526 Padua, Italy
e-mail: gianpaolo.rossi@unipd.it

G. Mancia (ed.), *Resistant Hypertension*, DOI: 10.1007/978-88-470-5415-8_2,

Table 2.1 Conditions and neurohumoral factors that can lead to "resistant hypertension"

• Activation of the renin–angiotensin system
- Renovascular hypertension
- Renin-secreting tumor
• Excess mineralocorticoid receptor activation
- Primary aldosteronism
- Apparent mineralocorticoid excess
• Miscellanea
- Obstructive sleep apnea syndrome
• Excess glucocorticoid activity
- Cushing syndrome
• Excess catecholamines effect
- Pheochromocytoma

The two most common renovascular diseases are fibromuscular dysplasia and atherosclerosis. Fibromuscular dysplasia accounts for less than one-fifth of the RVH patients at referral centers and occurs typically in young females where it usually affects the mid-portion of the renal artery [1]. It responds well to percutaneous transluminal renal angioplasty (PTRA) with long-term cure of high BP or at least with control of high BP.

Atherosclerotic plaques are usually an extension to the renal artery of a diffuse aorto-iliac disease, and therefore, they typically involve in the origin of the renal artery. Hence, the mean age of presentation of atherosclerotic RVH is over 50 years and two-thirds are men, with multiple CV risk factors and/or widespread atherosclerosis involving the carotid, the cerebrovascular, and the coronary arteries [1]. Because of its progressive nature, atherosclerotic renal artery stenosis induces renal atrophy in about one-fifth of patients in whom the stenosis was initially greater than 60 %. Moreover, due to its increasing prevalence with aging, it is becoming a leading cause of end-stage kidney disease.

The prevalence of RVH in the RH population is unknown, but experience indicates that the atherosclerotic form is increasingly recognized when properly searched for. It should be remembered, however, that the demonstration of a renal artery stenosis, albeit being a "must" for the diagnosis, does not fulfill *per se* a diagnosis of RVH because the renovascular disease can concur with primary high BP by chance and/or as a result of accelerated atherosclerosis. Proof of a cause–effect relationship between renal artery stenosis and RH can only be made retrospectively, when correction of renal ischemia controls or cures the high BP. This implies that endovascular treatment should be offered to all patients with RH and concomitant renal artery stenosis. In fact, RH ranks first among the clinical clues that suggest RVH, which include also onset of high BP before age 30 especially in females or after 50 especially in males, sudden onset or worsening of a previously controlled high BP, severe high BP with signs and/or symptoms of atherosclerosis, smoking, unexplained recurrent episodes of heart failure and/or pulmonary edema, abdominal (or femoral or carotid) systo-diastolic bruits, and stage II–IV Keith–Wagener–Barker retinopathy. Ultrasonographic, CT, or mineralocorticoid receptor (MR) evidence of atherosclerosis in other vascular beds and/or of a unilateral small kidney should also suggest RVH.

Hyperreninemia is held to be the hallmark of RVH but lacks in up to one-third of the cases, because overt activation of the renin–angiotensin–aldosterone system (RAAS) occurs only early on when the stenosis becomes hemodynamically relevant [2]. Later with time, however, the high BP and the stimulation of sodium reabsorption, resulting from the action angiotensin II and aldosterone on the renal tubule, blunt renin secretion. Moreover, the hypertrophic remodeling in small arteries (increased vessel wall-to-lumen ratio) enhances the pressor effect of angiotensin II, which explains why BP remains high in spite of normal or even low renin levels [2]. Thus, the chances of detecting hyperreninemia are high when the patient is seen soon after the onset of high BP, but diminish afterward, which explains why many patients with RH due to RVH do not have high renin at the time of diagnosis. Utmost care should be taken to the conditions under which measuring renin. This is because renin values are affected by posture, sodium intake, and drug therapy as discussed elsewhere in more detail [3], and therefore proper precautions are to be taken. Attention to concurrent treatment with antihypertensive drugs is particularly important in patients with RH in that it usually precludes a "clean" assessment of the RAAS. Hence, knowledge of the effect of each class of agents on the RAAS, as reported in Table 2.2 and discussed later, can assist in properly interpreting the renin (and aldosterone) levels. Concomitant treatment with beta-blockers and/or non-steroidal anti-inflammatory drugs blunts renin secretion, while ACE inhibitors, ARBs, and diuretics raise it. Moreover, hypokalemia raised serum creatinine levels and impaired glomerular filtration rate, proteinuria, and/or a sudden increase after ACE inhibition or AT1 receptor blockers should also alert on the possibility of RVH [3].

The ultimate test for diagnosing renovascular disease is selective renal angiography, which can provide a streamlined approach to percutaneous revascularization in patients with RH. However, at our institution, we generally prefer to undertake before a Doppler ultrasonography with measurement of the intrarenal resistive index (RI). The finding of homogeneously increased (>0.80) RI in the upper, middle, and lower third of each kidney suggests nephroangiosclerosis, while decreased values and/or the detection of within-kidney heterogeneity of RI values are clues to significant renal artery stenosis. We next proceed to performing an angio-CT or MR angiography to confirm the diagnosis and gather information that are useful for the planning of selective renal angiography aimed at percutaneous endovascular treatment.

The AHA guidelines recommend revascularization in patients with hemodynamically significant atherosclerotic renal artery stenosis, falling in the following categories: recurrent, unexplained CHF or sudden, unexplained pulmonary embolism (Class I recommendation, level of evidence: B); accelerated and/or resistant and/or malignant hypertension, hypertension with an unexplained

Table 2.2 Effects of drugs and conditions on the RAAS

Factor	PAC	Renin	ARR	False-positive rate	False-negative rate
Medications					
β blockers	↓	↓↓	↑	↑↑	↓
Central α-2 agonists	↓	↓↓	↑	↑	↓
NSAIDs	↓	↓↓	↑	↑	↓
K^+ losing diuretics	↑	↑↑	↓	↓	↑
K^+ sparing diuretics	↑	↑↑	↓	↓	↑
ACE inhibitors	↓	↑↑	↓	↓	↑
ARBs	↓	↑↑	↓	↓	↑
Long-acting CCBs	→↓	→	↓	→↓	→↑
Renin inhibitors	↓	↓↑*	↓*↑ *	↓*↑ *	↓*↑ *
Hypokalemia	↓	→↑	↓	↓	↑
Sodium depletion	↑	↑↑	↓	↓	↑
Sodium loading	↓	↓↓	↑	↑	↓
Aging	↓	↓↓	↑	↑	
Other conditions					
Renal impairment	→	↓	↑	↑	↓
Pregnancy	↑	↑↑	↓	↓	↓
Renovascular	↑	↑↑	↓	↓	↑

β blockers suppress renin but affect PAC relatively less, thus raising the ARR and the false-positive rate. Drugs that raise the PRA more than PAC, such as diuretics and MR antagonists, increase the rate of false-negative diagnoses. Angiotensin-converting enzyme (*ACE*) inhibitors, angiotensin II receptor blockers (*ARBs*), and renin inhibitors raise renin and reduce aldosterone secretion. Therefore, they reduce the ARR and increase the false-negative rate. *Renin inhibitors lower PRA but raise DRA. This effect would be expected to increase false positives when renin is measured as PRA, and false negatives for renin if measured as DRA. Abbreviations, ARR, aldosterone: renin ratio; DRA, direct active renin; PAC, plasma aldosterone concentration; PRA, plasma renin activity

unilateral small kidney and/or with intolerance to medication, progressive chronic kidney disease with bilateral renal artery stenosis or with a solitary functioning kidney, unstable angina (all with Class IIA recommendation, level of evidence: B); asymptomatic bilateral or solitary viable kidney, asymptomatic unilateral renal artery stenosis in a viable kidney, and chronic kidney disease with unilateral renal artery stenosis (all Class IIB recommendation, level of evidence: C) [4]. Due to the lack data from randomized clinical trials none of these indications reached Class I recommendation, level of evidence A.

2.3 Primary Reninism

Juxtaglomerular cell tumors secreting renin are very rare causes of surgically curable RH. Their clinical picture closely resembles RVH in that they entail prominent activation of the RAAS, usually with markedly increased renin levels, hyperaldosteronism, and hypokalemia. Most patients are young and present with severe, or sometimes malignant, high BP. The lack of renal artery stenosis and the finding of a lateralized renin secretion at renal vein renin studies mandate a CT or MR scan to search for a small kidney mass, whose identification can be difficult because even at angiography because of angiotensin II-induced vasoconstriction. Tumorectomy resolved RH provides relief from the secondary hyperaldosteronism [3].

2.4 Excess Mineralocorticoid Receptor Activation

In the tissues that are target of aldosterone, including the distal renal epithelial tubules, the blood vessels, and the heart, activation of the MR leads to increase in pre- and after load and to adverse CV changes, including hypertrophy and fibrosis, which ultimately cause CV events [5, 6]. In the last decade, compelling evidences have been provided that primary aldosteronism (PA) is the most common cause of arterial hypertension among the hypertensive patients referred to specialized hypertension centers. In the PAPY study, the largest prospective survey, the prevalence of PA was 11.2 % [7], and half of the cases were surgically curable.

The contention that RH has a high of PA remained based on anecdotal data until in 2005 a study from our group showed that 42 % of 157 patients referred to the outpatient clinic for RH had PA and the remaining 58 % responded well to MR antagonists [8], thus indicating the role of excess MR activation in causing resistance of BP to treatment. A much larger retrospective study thereafter showed that 20.9 % of 1,616 patients with RH had PA, as demonstrated by a raised aldosterone/renin ratio (ARR) and plasma aldosterone concentration [9]. Noteworthy, only 45.6 % of the patients with PA had hypokalemia. Thus, the conclusion can be drawn that (1) 11.2–42 % of the patients referred for RH patients with RH have PA; (2) hypokalemia lacks in the majority of the PA patients with RH and therefore should not be used as the "alerting" sign [10–12].

By definition, RH patients are on a multiple antihypertensive drug regimen at presentation, which can affect the PAC and renin values, and therefore, the ARR should be modified, if feasible, before measuring these hormones. Beta-blockers raise the ARR and should be stopped at least two weeks before the measurement of the PAC and renin [10]. Conversely, diuretics and MR antagonists should be withdrawn before 2 and 6 weeks, respectively, because they raise the PRA.

Angiotensin-converting enzyme (ACE) inhibitors and sartans (ARBs) have an even more marked effect not only because they raise the PRA, but also because they blunt aldosterone secretion, thus reducing the ARR and increasing false-negative results. Therefore, they should be withdrawn at least 2–3 weeks before performing the ARR. Other agents have no or minimal effects on the ARR: The α1-receptor blocker doxazosin does not affect the RAAS, while the short-acting calcium channel blockers (CCB) can blunt aldosterone secretion and raise the PRA and, therefore, can cause false-negative results; the long-acting CCB have a small blunting effect on aldosterone secretion [10, 12, 13]. However, the withdrawal of antihypertensive treatment is dangerous for the patients with RH, and therefore, they should be tested while on treatment, possibly with long-acting CCB and/or a α1-receptor blocker. If even this is unsafe, one should make use of the aforementioned theoretical notions on drug effect (Table 2.2) on these hormones.

It should also be recalled that sodium and water retention, an important factor contributing to RH, lowers renin. Hence, a low renin value is a sign of volume and sodium overload, and not necessarily a hint to the presence of PA. The measurement of estimated GFR and urinary sodium output can allow identifying this condition.

RH implies *per se* a higher likelihood of events, which can be amplified by PA [6, 11]. Thus, the diagnosis of PA should not be missed or delayed in patients with RH. Thus, the screening for PA can have a great impact on the life expectancy for the affected patients. As patients with RH are at increased risk and have a high (between 11 and 30 %) pretest probability of PA, the possibility of PA should be considered in all patients with RH.

There is little doubt that if the patients are not a reasonable candidate to general anesthesia or are not willing to undergo surgery, a MR antagonist should be added with a careful surveillance of renal function and serum K^+. Conversely, if the patient is a candidate for general anesthesia and adrenalectomy and seeks definitive cure, efforts should be devoted to identify a lateralized cause for aldosterone excess as described elsewhere [10].

If lateralized aldosterone excess has been demonstrated, laparoscopic adrenalectomy is the treatment of choice. It can be performed during a short hospital stay at a very low operative risk and provides cure of arterial hypertension in 30–40 % of the patients at long-term, a marked improvement in BP central in up to 60–90 % and cure of hyperaldosteronism in practically all [10, 14].

In patients without lateralized aldosterone excess, MR antagonists such as spironolactone, canrenone, potassium canrenoate, and eplerenone are the alternative to adrenalectomy. The occurrence of gynecomastia and impotence, which can occur with these agents, is dose-dependent, which suggests use of reduced doses administered in combination, if necessary, with other agents, such as long-acting CCBs, ACE inhibitors, or ARBs. ACE inhibitors and ARBs are particularly useful, as they effectively control the stimulation of the RAAS by the diuretic action of the MR antagonists [10].

2.5 Apparent Mineralocorticoid Excess

Apparent mineralocorticoid excess (AME) is a rare monogenic form of hypertension caused by the loss of the activity of 11 β-hydroxysteroid dehydrogenase type 2 (11 β-HSD2), an enzyme that colocalizes with the MR and inactivates cortisol to cortisone in the target tissues of aldosterone. Under normal conditions, this inactivation protects the receptor from cortisol binding, thus allowing aldosterone to gain access to its receptor. Several mutations of the HSD11B2 gene were found to blunt enzyme activity, resulting in cortisol-induced activation of the MR and in a clinical phenotype mimicking PA despite no aldosterone excess.

AME is inherited as an autosomal recessive trait and is characterized by a close genotype–phenotype correlation. Homozygous AME usually presents early in life with severe RH, hypokalemia, metabolic alkalosis, and low levels of renin and aldosterone. The biochemical diagnosis can be made by the demonstration of an increased (up to 33) ratio THF:THE, (normal values about 1) in a 24-h urine collection.

Subjects ingesting large amount of licorice or carbenoxolone can mimic AME, because of the inhibiting effect on 11 β-HSD2 and the (weak) mineralocorticoid activity of these substances.

2.6 Obstructive Sleep Apnea Syndrome

Obstructive sleep apnea syndrome (OSAS) is a common albeit under diagnosed cause of RH [15]. The patients are more often men, above 50, overweight or obese, with a history of smoking and/or COPD. Repeated episodes of desaturation during sleep are held to induce recurrent sympathetic activation, blunted catecholamines inactivation, increased synthesis of aldosterone [15] and of the potent vasoconstrictor endothelin-1, and blunted bioactivity of the vasodilator nitric oxide. Correction of repeated desaturation episodes by non-pharmacologic measures, surgery, or CPAP usually lowers BP and can resolve resistance to treatment.

2.7 Excess Glucocorticoid Activity

Cushing syndrome, both endogenous and, more commonly, iatrogenic, is usually self-evident and represents a very rare cause of RH. The diagnosis stands on the demonstration of excess cortisol in plasma, saliva, and urines [3].

2.8 Excess Catecholamines

The prevalence of catecholamine-secreting tumors as pheochromocytoma (Pheo) in patients presenting with RH is unknown, but probably very low. Due to the huge variation in its clinical presentation, with symptoms ranging from none to many,

Pheo has been defined as "the great simulator" [1, 3], which implies that no symptoms or signs are pathognomonic for the disease.

These diverse clinical manifestations reflect variations in the amount, type, and patterns of hormone release and in interindividual differences in catecholamines sensitivity. The most common norepinephrine (NE)-secreting Pheo is usually associated with sustained high BP, while those also secreting relatively large amounts of epinephrine (E) can be associated with episodic high BP [3]. Overall, BP is persistently high in only one-third of Pheo patients [3], which implies that the finding of normal catecholamine levels in a patient with RH makes the diagnosis of Pheo unlikely.

The high BP in Pheo has been attributed to the action of excess circulating catecholamines on CV adrenergic receptors, because the activity of the sympathetic nervous system would be either normal or depressed through baroreceptor resetting. Accordingly, neurally released NE would play a minor physiological role in comparison with the effects of markedly elevated plasma catecholamine levels. These assumptions are, however, untenable, because in patients with Pheo (1) BP values do not correlate with circulating catecholamines; (2) inhibition of neurally mediated catecholamine release (with clonidine) significantly reduced BP and heart rate despite leaving the high circulating catecholamines unaffected; (3) sympathetic reflexes are intact. Moreover, experimental studies collectively indicated that the sympathetic nervous system is markedly enhanced and that its function is crucial for the maintenance of high BP.

The excessive stores of NE in sympathetic nerve terminals, along with the enhanced sympathetic nervous system activity, imply that any direct or reflexly mediated stimulus to the sympathetic nervous system can trigger a hypertensive crisis via excess release of NE into the synaptic cleft. Hence, spontaneous or evoked hypertensive crises can arise without any increases in the elevated plasma catecholamine levels.

Other neurohormonal agents, including neuropeptide Y (NPY), chromogranin A, and adrenomedullin, contribute to the pathophysiology of Pheo and were reviewed elsewhere [1, 3].

Any RH patient with symptoms or signs even remotely suggestive of a Pheo should be considered for screening. This is because Pheo is a potentially fatal disease and therefore should be conclusively confirmed, or excluded, whenever the suspicion arises. Hence, a high degree of alert to the possibility of a Pheo should be exercised in RH patients, and an ultrasound investigation of the adrenals and assays of urine for metanephrines excretion are mandatory. Because of the deceptive and varied manifestations of Pheo, the optimal pretreatment evaluation stands on the demonstration of excessive and inappropriate production of catecholamines and other substances that are secreted by the tumor as described elsewhere [1]. However, one should bear in mind that the milestone for the diagnosis is clinical judgment and that laboratory testing should complement it and not replace it.

Recent studies have shown that mutations are not exclusive of the familial (hereditary) Pheo, but are found in about 25 % of the patients with apparently sporadic Pheo. Such patients should be tested for germline mutations if they are young, asymptomatic, and/or have multifocal tumors and extra-adrenal tumors, [16]. Finding a germline mutation is important not only for the patient's, but also for the relatives in that it will lead to surveillance and early diagnosis of the disease.

In patients with Pheo imaging, tests are required to locate the tumor, not the other way around, although the incidental discovery of Pheo often reverses the order. A detailed discussion of the techniques for the localization of Pheo is available elsewhere. Finally, it has to be remembered that malignant Pheo can be diagnosed because of metastasis as long as 15 years after successful surgical excision, which underscores the lack of good ways to diagnose malignancy and the need of follow-up.

The patients should be treated with doxazosin followed by β-blockers, not the way around, because blockade of β-adrenoceptor without previous α_1-adrenoceptor blockade can worsen the hypertension dramatically. Once adequately prepared, the patients should be referred for surgery, bearing in mind that follow-up is necessary to identify recurrences.

2.9 Conclusions

Activation of neurohumoralsystems is a common primary mechanism of resistance of high BP to drug treatment. RH patients are by definition on multiple antihypertensive drugs that cannot be withdrawn, which poses special diagnostic challenges. However, physicians should not be discouraged from embarking in the workup that is required to attain the diagnosis, as the identification of the underlying mechanism is rewarding in that it usually results in resolution of RH.

Acknowledgment The studies reported in this chapter were mostly supported by research grants from The FOundation for advanced Research In Hypertension and CArdiovascular diseases (FORICA), The Società Italiana dell'Ipertensione Arteriosa, The Italian Ministry of University and Scientific Research (MIUR), and The University of Padua.

References

1. Rossi GP, Seccia TM, Pessina AC (2010) Secondary hypertension: the ways of management. Curr Vasc Pharmacol 8:753–768
2. Rossi GP, Zanin L, Mazzucco B, De Toni R, Bader M, Chiesura-Corona M, Feltrin GP, Pessina AC (1997) Renovascular hypertension with low-to-normal plasma renin: clinical features, diagnostic and prognostic implications. Clin Sci 93:435–443
3. Rossi GP, Seccia TM, Pessina AC (2007) Clinical use of laboratory tests for the identification of secondary forms of arterial hypertension. Crit Rev Clin Lab Sci 44:1–85
4. Hirsch AT, Haskal ZJ, Hertzer NR, Bakal CW, Creager MA, Halperin JL, Hiratzka LF, Murphy WR, Olin JW, Puschett JB, Rosenfield KA, Sacks D, Stanley JC, Taylor LM Jr,

White CJ, White J, White RA, Antman EM, Smith SC Jr, Adams CD, Anderson JL, Faxon DP, Fuster V, Gibbons RJ, Hunt SA, Jacobs AK, Nishimura R, Ornato JP, Page RL, Riegel B (2006) American Association for Vascular Surgery; Society for Vascular Surgery; Society for Cardiovascular Angiography and Interventions; Society for Vascular Medicine and Biology; Society of Interventional Radiology; ACC/AHA Task Force on Practice Guidelines Writing Committee to Develop Guidelines for the Management of Patients With Peripheral Arterial Disease; American Association of Cardiovascular and Pulmonary Rehabilitation; National Heart, Lung, and Blood Institute; Society for Vascular Nursing; Transatlantic Inter-Society Consensus; Vascular Disease Foundation. ACC/AHA 2005 Practice Guidelines for the management of patients with peripheral arterial disease (lower extremity, renal, mesenteric, and abdominal aortic): a collaborative report from the American Association for Vascular Surgery/Society for Vascular Surgery, Society for Cardiovascular Angiography and Interventions, Society for Vascular Medicine and Biology, Society of Interventional Radiology, and the ACC/AHA Task Force on Practice Guidelines (Writing Committee to Develop Guidelines for the Management of Patients With Peripheral Arterial Disease): endorsed by the American Association of Cardiovascular and Pulmonary Rehabilitation; National Heart, Lung, and Blood Institute; Society for Vascular Nursing; Transatlantic Inter-Society Consensus; and Vascular Disease Foundation. Circulation 113(11):e463–654
5. Rossi GP, Pessina AC, Heagerty AM (2008) Primary aldosteronism: an update on screening, diagnosis and treatment. J Hypertens 26:613–621
6. Rossi GP, Sechi LA, Giacchetti G, Ronconi V, Strazzullo P, Funder JW (2008) Primary aldosteronism: cardiovascular, renal and metabolic implications. Trends Endocrinol Metab 19:88–90
7. Rossi GP, Bernini G, Caliumi C, Desideri G, Fabris B, Ferri C, Ganzaroli C, Giacchetti G, Letizia C, Maccario M, Mallamaci F, Mannelli M, Mattarello MJ, Moretti A, Palumbo G, Parenti G, Porteri E, Semplicini A, Rizzoni D, Rossi E, Boscaro M, Pessina AC, Mantero F (2006) A prospective study of the prevalence of primary aldosteronism in 1,125 hypertensive patients. J Am Coll Cardiol 48:2293–2300
8. Sartori M, Calo LA, Mascagna V, Realdi A, Macchini L, Ciccariello L et al (2006) Aldosterone and refractory hypertension: a prospective cohort study. Am J Hypertens 19:373–379
9. Douma S, Petidis K, Doumas M, Papaefthimiou P, Triantafyllou A, Kartali N, Papadopoulos N, Vogiatzis K, Zamboulis C (2008) Prevalence of primary hyperaldosteronism in resistant hypertension: a retrospective observational study. Lancet 7(371):1921–1926
10. Rossi GP (2011) A comprehensive review of the clinical aspects of primary aldosteronism. Nat Rev Endocrinol 24(7):485–495
11. Calhoun DA, Nishizaka MK, Zaman MA, Thakkar RB, Weissmann P (2002) Hyperaldosteronism among black and white subjects with resistant hypertension. Hypertension 40:892–896
12. Funder JW, Carey RM, Fardella C, Gomez-Sanchez CE, Mantero F, Stowasser M, Young WF Jr, Montori VM (2008) Case detection, diagnosis, and treatment of patients with primary aldosteronism: an endocrine society clinical practice guideline. J Clin Endocrinol Metab 93:3266–3281
13. Mulatero P, Rabbia F, Milan A, Paglieri C, Morello F, Chiandussi L, Veglio F (2002) Drug effects on aldosterone/plasma renin activity ratio in primary aldosteronism. Hypertension 40:897–902
14. Rossi GP, Bolognesi M, Rizzoni D, Seccia TM, Piva A, Porteri E, Tiberio GA, Giulini SM, Agabiti-Rosei E, Pessina AC (2008) Vascular remodeling and duration of hypertension predict outcome of adrenalectomy in primary aldosteronism patients. Hypertension 51:1366–1371
15. Goodfriend TL, Calhoun DA (2004) Resistant hypertension, obesity, sleep apnea, and aldosterone: theory and therapy. Hypertension 43:518–524

16. Neumann HP, Bausch B, McWhinney SR, Bender BU, Gimm O, Franke G, Schipper J, Klisch J, Altehoefer C, Zerres K, Januszewicz A, Eng C, Smith WM, Munk R, Manz T, Glaesker S, Apel TW, Treier M, Reineke M, Walz MK, Hoang-Vu C, Brauckhoff M, Klein-Franke A, Klose P, Schmidt H, Maier-Woelfle M, Peçzkowska M, Szmigielski C, Eng C (2002) Freiburg-Warsaw-Columbus Pheochromocytoma Study Group Germ-line mutations in nonsyndromic pheochromocytoma. N Engl J Med 346:1459–1466

3 Metabolic Alterations

Christian Delles and Anna F. Dominiczak

3.1 Introduction

The prevalence of obesity is steadily increasing in Western societies, and currently about a third of the US population are obese [1]. Similarly, hypertension is a worldwide phenomenon that affects both developed and developing countries, and about a quarter of the world's population has elevated blood pressure [2]. If two highly prevalent conditions co-exist, it is very likely that many patients are affected by both. In addition to the statistical odds, there are, however, also causal relationships between metabolic disorders, obesity, and hypertension [3]. These pathophysiological mechanisms and their implications on patients with hypertension will be the subject of this chapter (Fig. 3.1).

The epidemiological and pathophysiological links between blood pressure and obesity have led to the inclusion of hypertension as one of the factors of the metabolic syndrome (Table 3.1). Although some authors argue that hypertension is "less metabolic" than other factors such as dyslipidemia and impaired glucose tolerance [4], it is evident that hypertension is one of the major complications of obesity and contributes to the high cardiovascular risk of obese people [3]. In addition, obesity further aggravates hypertension and affects adversely the response to antihypertensive treatment. In a seminal paper, Modan et al. [5] demonstrated a direct relationship between body mass index (BMI) and the number of antihypertensive drugs that are required to control blood pressure. Independent of BMI itself, the number of antihypertensive drugs in this study was

C. Delles · A. F. Dominiczak (✉)
Institute of Cardiovascular and Medical Sciences, University of Glasgow,
126 University Place, Glasgow, G12 8TA, UK
e-mail: Anna.Dominiczak@glasgow.ac.uk

C. Delles
e-mail: Christian.Delles@glasgow.ac.uk

G. Mancia (ed.), *Resistant Hypertension*, DOI: 10.1007/978-88-470-5415-8_3,

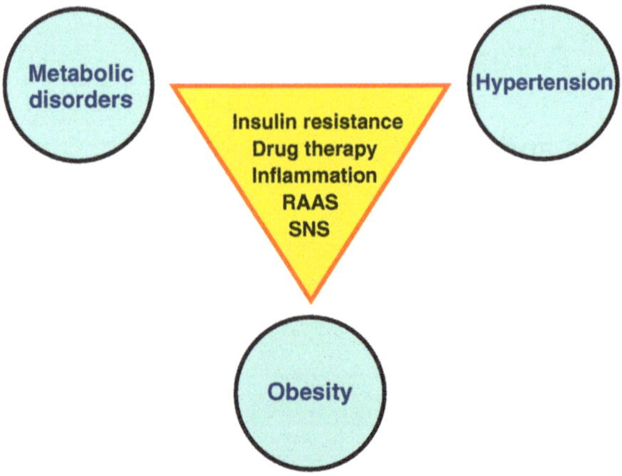

Fig. 3.1 Interaction between hypertension, obesity, and metabolic disorders. Shared pathogenetic factors include insulin resistance, activation of the sympathetic nervous system (*SNS*), and the renin–angiotensin–aldosterone system (*RAAS*), inflammation and the consequences of drug therapy

Table 3.1 Definitions of the metabolic syndrome

International Diabetes Federation
Central obesity and any two of the following:
• Raised triglycerides: >150 mg/dL (1.7 mmol/L), or specific treatment for this lipid abnormality
• Reduced HDL cholesterol: <40 mg/dL (1.03 mmol/L) in males, <50 mg/dL (1.29 mmol/L) in females, or specific treatment for this lipid abnormality
• Raised blood pressure: systolic BP > 130 or diastolic BP > 85 mmHg, or treatment of previously diagnosed hypertension
• Raised fasting plasma glucose: >100 mg/dL (5.6 mmol/L), or previously diagnosed type 2 diabetes
World Health Organization
Any one of diabetes mellitus, impaired glucose tolerance, impaired fasting glucose or insulin resistance, and two of the following:
• Blood pressure: ≥140/90 mmHg
• Dyslipidemia: triglycerides: ≥150 mg/dL (1.7 mmol/L) and HDL cholesterol ≤35 mg/dL (0.9 mmol/L) (male), ≤39 mg/dL (1.0 mmol/L) (female)
• Central obesity: waist: hip ratio >0.90 (male); >0.85 (female), or body mass index >30 kg/m^2
• Microalbuminuria: urinary albumin excretion ratio ≥20 μg/min or albumin:creatinine ratio ≥30 mg/g
US National Cholesterol Education Program Adult Treatment Panel III
At least three of the following:
• Central obesity: waist circumference ≥102 cm (40 in) (male), ≥88 cm (36 in) (female)

(continued)

Table 3.1 (continued)

• Dyslipidemia: triglycerides ≥150 mg/dl (1.7 mmol/L)
• Dyslipidemia: HDL cholesterol <40 mg/dL (1.0 mmol/L) (male), <50 mg/dL (1.3 mmol/L) (female)
• Blood pressure ≥130/85 mmHg
• Fasting plasma glucose ≥110 mg/dL (6.1 mmol/L)

The International Diabetes Federation definition recommends an oral glucose tolerance test if fasting plasma glucose is >100 mg/dL (5.6 mmol/L) and assumes central obesity if BMI >30 kg/m^2. Further details on these definitions are provided in [57]

also associated with glucose tolerance and hyperinsulinemia, suggesting that these metabolic alterations may provide the mechanistic link between hypertension and obesity [5]. It follows directly from these considerations that metabolic disorders and obesity are particularly prevalent in patients with resistant hypertension. Along the same lines, presence of the metabolic syndrome significantly increases cardiovascular risk in patients with hypertension (Fig. 3.2).

In this chapter, we will highlight some aspects of the relationship between metabolic disorders and hypertension. We will briefly review the epidemiologic and genetic links between the conditions, discuss some of the pathophysiological

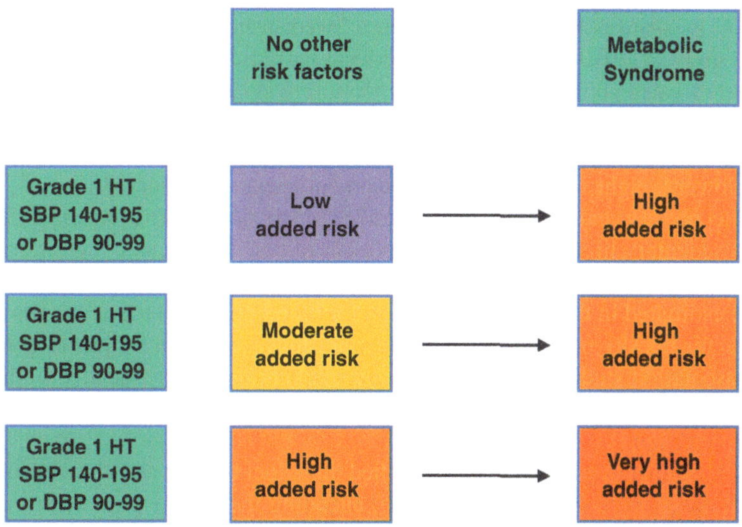

Fig. 3.2 Cardiovascular risk associated with the metabolic syndrome. The figure focuses on patients with resistant hypertension who, by definition, have blood pressure above 140/90 mmHg despite treatment with at least three drug classes including a diuretic. Presence of the metabolic syndrome increases cardiovascular risk significantly. Note that this chart is only an approximation as it does not accurately show cardiovascular risk in resistant hypertension but in grade 1, 2, and 3 hypertension (HT). Modified from [42]

mechanisms, and then examine the implications of metabolic disorders on the treatment of patients with hypertension.

3.2 Obesity and Hypertension: Epidemiological and Genetic Aspects

According to the National Health and Nutrition Examination Survey (NHANES), the prevalence of obesity in the United States was 32.2 % among adult men and 35.5 % among women in 2007–2008 [1]. Although the prevalence of obesity in women has not changed significantly over a 10-year observation period and the rate appears to increase more slowly recently in men, the overall prevalence of obesity is alarmingly high. In the Framingham Offspring Study, adiposity as assessed by subscapular skinfold has been found to the major controllable contributor to hypertension [6]. The role of obesity in the development has been confirmed in other longitudinal studies including the Atherosclerosis Risk in Communities Study in 9,309 white and African-American men and women; weight gain over the 6-year follow-up period was associated with increased blood pressure and increased incidence of hypertension [7]. Conversely, weight loss has been found to be associated with reduction in blood pressure in the Nurses' Health Study where long-term weight loss in women after the age of 18 years reduced the risk of hypertension with relative risks of 0.85 and 0.74 for a weight loss of 5–9.9 kg and ≥10 kg, respectively [8]. In contrast, the effect of bariatric surgery on blood pressure is less pronounced. In a Swedish non-randomized 10-year follow-up study of 2,010 patients who underwent bariatric surgery and 2,037 controls who were treated conservatively, blood pressure was different between the groups at the 2-year follow-up visit, but there was no difference in blood pressure and incidence of hypertension between the groups at 10 years—despite the significantly lower weight in patients who underwent bariatric surgery [9].

While obesity and hypertension share common causal environmental factors such as sedentary lifestyle, it is also important to note that genetic factors account for both conditions. Heritabilities have been assessed from family and twin studies and are estimated in the range of 15–40 % for blood pressure [10] and in the range of 40 % for obesity measures [11]. Both conditions have been subject to genome-wide association studies (GWAS). Genetic markers that are associated with both conditions may provide further explanations for the causal links between obesity and hypertension.

A GWAS in adolescent obesity identified three loci that are associated with both total fat mass and blood pressure: *PAX5*, encoding the transcription factor paired box protein Pax-5; *MRPS22*, encoding the mitochondrial ribosomal protein S22; and *FTO*, encoding the mRNA demethylase Fat mass and obesity-associated protein [12]. In a French Canadian founder population, the potential role of *FTO* to mediate both obesity and hypertension was confirmed and a role of the gene product in modulating sympathetic activity has been proposed [13]. In a genome-wide linkage study into obesity-associated hypertension in 55 French Canadian families, loci on chromosomes 1 and 11 were identified that contain promising candidates including tumor necrosis factor receptor 2 and atrial natriuretic peptide genes [14]. In a recent GWAS in 200,000 individuals of European descent, a polymorphism in the *SLC39A8* gene that has previously been described as being associated with BMI [15] has also been found to be associated with blood pressure [16]. *SLC39A8* encodes a zinc transporter that is critical in the defences against inflammation and oxidative stress. In summary, these studies provide evidence that obesity and hypertension have common genetic determinants, but further functional dissection of these signals is required.

3.3 Pathogenetic Links Between Obesity and Hypertension

3.3.1 Adipose Tissue

Adipose tissue, and in particular the visceral adipose tissue (VAT), produces a number of factors that directly or indirectly affect vascular function and structure [17, 18]. Such adipokines include angiotensin II and endothelin-1, which cause direct vasoconstriction; renin, which can be taken up by vascular tissue to catalyze the conversion of angiotensinogen to angiotensin I [19]; and non-esterified fatty acids (NEFA) which have been found to impair vascular nitric oxide production and thereby cause endothelial dysfunction [20]. In addition, macrophage infiltration in adipose tissue leads to further release of proinflammatory cytokines such as interleukin-6 with subsequent initiation of acute-phase responses, changes in vascular function and initiation of atherosclerosis [21].

Apart from the systemic release of adipokines through VAT, there are more local effects of specific adipose tissue on the vasculature. For example, the epicardial adipose tissue (EAT) is thought to contribute to local oxidative stress due to reduced expression of the antioxidant enzyme catalase compared to VAT. This phenomenon has been found to be associated with atherosclerosis in nearby coronary vessels [22]. The most direct effect of visceral tissue on vascular function is seen in the interaction between perivascular adipose tissue (PVAT) and blood vessels [17]. Healthy PVAT has anticontractile properties probably through actions of adiponectin, leptin, and angiotensin 1–7. In obesity, there is disruption of these anticontractile properties, triggered by macrophage infiltration, release of proinflammatory cytokines such as TNF-alpha and interleukin-6, and increased levels of reactive oxygen species [23].

3.3.2 Insulin Resistance

A key feature of obesity and the metabolic syndrome is insulin resistance. There is evidence that the close links between hypertension and the metabolic syndrome are due to hypertension being an insulin-resistant state [24]. The cellular disturbances in insulin-resistant states are characterized by changes in glucose and lipid metabolism that are associated with the generation of reactive oxygen species. These in turn reduce the bioavailability of the vasodilator nitric oxide and thereby cause endothelial dysfunction. The high insulin levels that characterize obesity and early stages of type 2 diabetes can therefore explain at least in part the endothelial dysfunction in these people [25].

3.3.3 Lipids

Dyslipidemia is one of the cardinal features of the metabolic syndrome. Hypercholesterolemia has been shown to be associated with endothelial dysfunction in various vascular systems including the coronary, forearm, and renal circulation. There is a quantitative inverse relationship between LDL cholesterol levels and endothelium-dependent vasodilation, and between triglyceride levels and endothelium-dependent vasodilation [26]. Endothelial dysfunction is an early characteristic of any vascular disease and ultimately leads to hypertension and associated organ damage [27].

It is therefore not unreasonable to speculate that lipid-lowering therapy could lead to a reduction in blood pressure. Data from a number of smaller studies [28] but also from a large (n = 973) clinical trial [29] suggest a modest blood pressure–lowering effect of statins. Unfortunately, the largest study on lipid-lowering therapy in hypertensive subjects, the lipid-lowering arm of the Anglo-Scandinavian Cardiac Outcomes Trial (ASCOT), was not able to provide data on a direct blood pressure-lowering effect of atorvastatin [30]. From the same study, it is evident, however, that atorvastatin, led to significant risk reduction in patients with hypertension. Global cardiovascular risk management including prescription of statins is therefore recommended in patients with hypertension, and in particular in those with the metabolic syndrome and/or resistant hypertension, but their specific blood pressure-lowering effect requires further studies [31].

3.3.4 Sympathetic Nervous System

Activation of the sympathetic nervous system is one of the hallmarks of obesity and the metabolic syndrome [32]. The sympathetic nervous system provides one of the links between blood pressure and insulin resistance in hypertensive subjects [33]. There is indeed evidence that reduction in central sympathetic outflow by the imidazoline derivative moxonidine improves not only blood pressure but also improves insulin sensitivity in a rat model of hypertension [34] and small clinical studies.

More recently, a catheter-based method for renal sympathetic nerve ablation has been introduced that reduces blood pressure [32]. This novel therapy is currently restricted to patients with severe and/or resistant hypertension, and it was therefore a logical step to study the metabolic effects of this treatment in these patients. Mahfoud et al. [35] demonstrated in a small pilot study that renal denervation is paralleled by reductions in the numbers of patients with diabetes, impaired fasting glucose and/or impaired glucose tolerance and an increase in the number of patients with normal glucose tolerance. It is too early to make any firm recommendations on the basis of this pilot study, and certainly renal denervation should not currently be considered in patients who do not have severe or resistant hypertension. However, due to the apparently excellent tolerability of renal denervation, applications outwith a primarily blood pressure-lowering indication may be considered in the future.

3.3.5 Renin–Angiotensin–Aldosterone System

The renin–angiotensin–aldosterone system (RAAS) is activated in obesity. Reasons for this activation include compression of the kidneys by intrarenal fat deposits and the presence of RAAS components in adipocytes [17, 36]. Of particular interest is aldosterone whose levels are also elevated in obesity and which causes sodium and fluid retention, vascular and cardiac fibrosis and stimulates the generation of vascular reactive oxygen species which in turn lead to reduced nitric oxide availability and endothelial dysfunction. Very recent work by Briones et al. [37] provides evidence for a putative direct link between obesity, the RAAS, and vascular dysfunction by demonstrating aldosterone production in adipocytes through calcineurin-dependent signaling pathways.

3.3.6 Polycystic Ovary Syndrome

The polycystic ovary syndrome (PCOS) affects up to 10 % of women of reproductive age. The syndrome is characterized by polycystic ovaries, irregularities of the menstrual cycle, and androgen excess. Remarkably, about a third of women with PCOS also fulfill the criteria for metabolic syndrome [38] and are in particular affected by obesity and hypertension. The exact mechanisms for hypertension in these women are not known and include increased androgen levels, activation of a local ovarian RAAS and release of endothelin-1 from ovaries [39, 40], but the association of hypertension with obesity in these women is intriguing. In line with other hypertensive disorders associated with obesity, treatment includes lifestyle modifications and diet. Blockade of the RAAS appears a logical first-line antihypertensive therapy, also because of a possible antiandrogenic effect of ACE inhibitors [41], although the child-bearing age of women with PCOS and possible teratogenic effects of RAAS blockade should be taken into account.

3.4 Effects of Drug Therapy

In the current ESH/ESC guidelines, there are five classes of antihypertensive drugs that are recommended as first-line therapeutic agents: angiotensin-converting enzyme inhibitors, angiotensin receptor blockers, beta receptor blockers, calcium channel blockers, and diuretics [42]. It should be noted that there are other international and country-specific guidelines with slightly different recommendations. In the British NICE/BHS guidelines, for example, beta blockers do not feature as first-line agents any more [NICE. Hypertension: clinical management of primary hypertension in adults. Clinical guideline CG127. http://guidance.nice.org.uk/CG127; Accessed 20 Apr 2013]. Nevertheless, the ESH/ESC guidelines provide robust recommendations for treatment of hypertension and take metabolic aspects into account [42, 43].

While all first-line agents have similar blood pressure-lowering effects and safety profiles, there are differences in their additional benefits but also in their adverse effects in certain conditions. Antihypertensive agents have direct and indirect effects on metabolic parameters that will be outlined in this section (Table 3.2). It should be noted, however, that in the treatment of patients with hypertension, blood pressure reduction is by far the most important aim, and to a

Table 3.2 Effects of antihypertensive agents on insulin resistance

Drug class	Effect on insulin resistance	Proposed mechanism(s)
ACE inhibitors	↓	Counteracting adipose tissue–derived angiotensin II
Angiotensin II receptor blockers	↓	Counteracting adipose tissue–derived angiotensin II PPAR-γ receptor agonism (telmisartan only)
Mineralocorticoid receptor antagonists	↓	Counteracting adipose tissue–derived aldosterone
Calcium channel blockers	↔	
Alpha-adrenoceptor antagonists	(↓)	Improvement of the decreased glucose disposal rate associated with hypertension Additional mild improvement of the lipid profile
Thiazide diuretics	↑	Reduction in pancreatic insulin secretion
Beta receptor blockers	↑	Several mechanisms proposed, including reduced insulin secretion and increased hepatic glucose production
Centrally acting antihypertensive agents	(↓)	Reduction in sympathetic nervous activity

Arrows indicate increased (↑) and reduced insulin resistance (↓) and neutral effects (↔) as a result of treatment with these agents. Centrally acting antihypertensive agents include clonidine, alpha-methyldopa, and imidazoline receptor–binding agents degree even adverse metabolic profiles can be accepted if significant blood pressure reduction can be achieved. In the treatment of patients with resistant hypertension, combinations of several agents including second-line options are often required so that their metabolic profiles cannot always be taken into account.

3.4.1 First-Line Antihypertensive Agents

Thiazide diuretics are important first-line antihypertensive agents. Especially in resistant hypertension, diuretics play a crucial role, and the condition is typically only defined if there is also resistance to sufficient doses of diuretics. Thiazides, however, reduce insulin sensitivity and have been associated with increased incidence of diabetes [44]. There is general agreement that high-dose thiazides should be avoided but that this drug class still has invaluable benefits for the treatment of hypertension. The combination of thiazide diuretics with other agents with a more favorite metabolic profile (e.g., angiotensin receptor blockers) may offset some of their unwanted metabolic effects.

Beta blockers also have an adverse metabolic effect that is characterized by reduction in insulin sensitivity and increased incidence of new-onset diabetes [45]. A number of other issues including less pronounced antihypertensive effects, weaker protection against target organ damage, and adverse effects on central as opposed to peripheral blood pressure have led to recommendations by some guidelines including the British NICE guidelines to remove beta blockers from the list of first-line agents. Again, this may be appropriate for therapy of uncomplicated hypertension with one or two agents. In patients with resistant hypertension, a combination of several agents is required to reduce blood pressure. A critical appraisal of the ESH/ESC guidelines provides more details on the discussion about beta blockers and concludes that their overall safety profiles are not necessarily worse than that of other antihypertensive agents [46].

Calcium channel blockers are generally considered metabolic neutral. This is particularly true for the modern longer-acting agents and long-term release preparations of the older, short-acting agents. Due to their generally low adverse effect rates and absence of requirements to monitor electrolytes or the ECG, calcium channel blockers are often a cornerstone of antihypertensive treatment, particularly in patients with resistant hypertension.

Angiotensin-converting enzyme inhibitors and *angiotensin receptor blockers* block the production of angiotensin II or directly inhibit its actions on the AT_1-receptor, respectively. Especially, direct receptor blockade counteracts the effects of adipose tissue–derived angiotensin II and may therefore have additional advantages in the treatment of patients with the metabolic syndrome. It has further been argued that within the class of angiotensin receptor blockers, telmisartan may be particularly beneficial in patients with the metabolic syndrome due to its action as a partial peroxisome proliferator-activated receptor-gamma receptor agonist which will lead to increased insulin sensitivity [47]. In the Ongoing Telmisartan Alone and in Combination with Ramipril Global Endpoint Trial (ONTARGET) and Telmisartan Randomized Assessment Study in ACE Intolerant Subjects with Cardiovascular Disease (TRANSCEND) trials with telmisartan, the adverse effect of impaired glucose tolerance on cardiovascular outcomes was confirmed [48]. However, the incidence of new-onset diabetes was similar between the ramipril and telmisartan arms in the ONTARGET trial [49] and in TRANSCEND [50] although in the latter, there was a trend toward lower incidence of diabetes in the telmisartan compared to the placebo arm ($P = 0.08$).

In summary, there are data to support beneficial metabolic effects of angiotensin-converting enzyme inhibitors and angiotensin receptor blockers, neutral effects of calcium channel blockers, and potentially adverse effects of thiazide diuretics and beta blockers. While these effects should be considered, the most important aim remains blood pressure control for which the evidence base is by far more robust than evidence of adverse cardiovascular outcomes due to adverse metabolic effects of some antihypertensive agents. Where possible, however, a combination of thiazides and beta blockers should be avoided particularly in patients with the metabolic syndrome [43].

3.4.2 Other Antihypertensive Agents

In the treatment of patients with resistant hypertension, physicians will often use second and third line antihypertensive agents to control blood pressure. We will highlight a few of these agents and their metabolic profile.

Doxazosin is a widely used alpha-1 receptor blocker with modest effect on blood pressure. It has mild beneficial effects on insulin resistance and has also been shown to improve lipid profiles [51]. In an euglycaemic clamp study, it was demonstrated that doxazosin improves the decreased glucose disposal rate associated with hypertension [52]. It is therefore certainly a suitable add-on therapeutic agent in patients with resistant hypertension especially if they also have the metabolic syndrome.

Centrally acting antihypertensive drugs such as alpha-methyldopa and the imidazoline receptor–binding agents moxonidine and rilmenidine reduce sympathetic nerve activity and are therefore expected to have a beneficial metabolic profile. Reduced insulin resistance as a result of treatment with centrally acting antihypertensive drugs has indeed been shown, and evidence from smaller studies is accumulating that the relatively well-tolerated moxonidine may be of particular use for the treatment of hypertensive patients with the metabolic syndrome [53].

The *mineralocorticoid receptor antagonists* spironolactone and eplerenone are key compounds in the treatment of resistant hypertension. Excess aldosterone levels are involved in the pathogenesis of insulin resistance, and insulin sensitivity improves after adrenalectomy and mineralocorticoid receptor blockade in patients with aldosterone-producing tumors [54]. Mineralocorticoid receptor antagonists therefore directly target the obesity-related vascular dysfunction which contributes to their blood pressure-lowering effects particularly in patients with resistant hypertension.

Despite the positive metabolic effects of some of these agents, the evidence base for long-term beneficial effects is less robust than for first-line agents. The recommendation to try and treat blood pressure to target also in resistant hypertension with first-line agents remains, but the metabolic profiles of first-line and other agents should be taken into account to tailor treatment individually to these patients.

3.4.3 Antihypertensive Effects of Lipid- and Glucose-Lowering Therapy

There is also some evidence of an antihypertensive effect of drugs that are used to treat dyslipidemia and diabetes. The modest antihypertensive effect of statins has been mentioned above. Similar data exist for antidiabetic drugs. A study in spontaneously hypertensive rats demonstrates direct vascular effects of metformin with significantly reduced blood pressure after a 4-week treatment period [55]. In the same rat model, peroxisome proliferator-activated receptor-beta activation with GW0742 also reduced blood pressure in a 5-week experiment [56]. These studies are small and there is limited backup from human trials. Nevertheless, it is not unreasonable to believe that better control of the metabolic syndrome will be associated with better blood pressure control.

3.5 Conclusions

Resistant hypertension and the metabolic syndrome are pathophysiologically related with each other and therefore often co-exist in the same patient. There are few trials specifically into treatment of resistant hypertension, and similarly few data exist on the cardiovascular consequences of treatment-induced metabolic changes or the cardiovascular benefits of treating metabolic features in patients with resistant hypertension. It appears reasonable, however, from an antihypertensive point of view to primarily focus on optimal blood pressure control and from a metabolic point of view to primarily focus on optimal treatment of dyslipidemia, diabetes, and obesity. Any synergistic effects of drug classes to treat one of these conditions on other conditions can be used to the patients' advantage.

Metabolically neutral or beneficial antihypertensive first-line agents such as angiotensin receptor blockers, angiotensin-converting enzyme inhibitors, and calcium channel blockers can be supplemented by other antihypertensive agents with similar metabolic profiles such as alpha-adrenergic receptor agonists, imidazoline receptor–binding drugs, and mineralocorticoid receptor antagonists. Combination with drugs with a less favorable metabolic profile including thiazide diuretics and beta blockers is often required to achieve acceptable blood pressure control. Selected patients may also benefit from novel treatment strategies such as renal denervation. There is evidence that treatment of metabolic parameters including insulin resistance and dyslipidemia improves vascular function and may even have modest additional antihypertensive effects.

The key role of obesity in the initiation of the metabolic syndrome but also in the pathophysiology of hypertension and particularly of resistant hypertension cannot be over-emphasized. Tackling the worldwide obesity epidemic is one of the most important health care issues that will reduce the number of patients with resistant hypertension and related adverse cardiovascular events.

References

1. Flegal KM, Carroll MD, Ogden CL, Curtin LR (2010) Prevalence and trends in obesity among US adults, 1999–2008. JAMA 303(3):235–241
2. Kearney PM, Whelton M, Reynolds K, Muntner P, Whelton PK, He J (2005) Global burden of hypertension: analysis of worldwide data. Lancet 365(9455):217–223
3. Malnick SD, Knobler H (2006) The medical complications of obesity. QJM 99(9):565–579
4. Grundy SM, Brewer HB Jr, Cleeman JI, Smith SC Jr, Lenfant C (2004) Definition of metabolic syndrome: report of the National heart, lung, and blood institute/American heart association conference on scientific issues related to definition. Arterioscler Thromb Vasc Biol 24(2):e13–e18
5. Modan M, Almog S, Fuchs Z, Chetrit A, Lusky A, Halkin H (1991) Obesity, glucose intolerance, hyperinsulinemia, and response to antihypertensive drugs. Hypertension 17(4):565–573
6. Garrison RJ, Kannel WB, Stokes J III, Castelli WP (1987) Incidence and precursors of hypertension in young adults: the Framingham offspring study. Prev Med 16(2):235–251
7. Stevens J, Chambless LE, Tyroler HA, Rosamond W, Nieto FJ et al (2002) Associations between weight gain and incident hypertension in a bi-ethnic cohort: the atherosclerosis risk in communities study. Int J Obes Relat Metab Disord 26(1):58–64
8. Huang Z, Willett WC, Manson JE, Rosner B, Stampfer MJ, Speizer FE et al (1998) Body weight, weight change, and risk for hypertension in women. Ann Intern Med 128(2):81–88
9. Sjostrom L, Lindroos AK, Peltonen M, Torgerson J, Bouchard C, Carlsson B et al (2004) Lifestyle, diabetes, and cardiovascular risk factors 10 years after bariatric surgery. N Engl J Med 351(26):2683–2693
10. Delles C, Padmanabhan S (2012) Genetics and hypertension: is it time to change my practice? Can J Cardiol 28(3):296–304
11. Pausova Z, Gossard F, Gaudet D, Tremblay J, Kotchen TA, Cowley AW et al (2001) Heritability estimates of obesity measures in siblings with and without hypertension. Hypertension 38(1):41–47
12. Melka MG, Bernard M, Mahboubi A, Abrahamowicz M, Paterson AD, Syme C et al (2012) Genome-wide scan for loci of adolescent obesity and their relationship with blood pressure. J Clin Endocrinol Metab 97(1):E145–E150
13. Pausova Z, Syme C, Abrahamowicz M, Xiao Y, Leonard GT, Perron M et al (2009) A common variant of the FTO gene is associated with not only increased adiposity but also elevated blood pressure in French Canadians. Circ Cardiovasc Genet 2(3):260–269
14. Pausova Z, Gaudet D, Gossard F, Bernard M, Kaldunski ML, Jomphe M et al (2005) Genome-wide scan for linkage to obesity-associated hypertension in French Canadians. Hypertension 46(6):1280–1285
15. Speliotes EK, Willer CJ, Berndt SI, Monda KL, Thorleifsson G, Jackson AU et al (2010) Association analyses of 249,796 individuals reveal 18 new loci associated with body mass index. Nat Genet 42(11):937–948
16. Ehret GB, Munroe PB, Rice KM, Bochud M, Johnson AD, Chasman DI et al (2011) Genetic variants in novel pathways influence blood pressure and cardiovascular disease risk. Nature 478(7367):103–109

17. Aghamohammadzadeh R, Heagerty AM (2012) Obesity-related hypertension: epidemiology, pathophysiology, treatments, and the contribution of perivascular adipose tissue. Ann Med 44(Suppl 1):S74–S84
18. Chaudhary K, Buddineni JP, Nistala R, Whaley-Connell A (2011) Resistant hypertension in the high-risk metabolic patient. Curr Diab Rep 11(1):41–46
19. Muller DN, Hilgers KF, Bohlender J, Lippoldt A, Wagner J, Fischli W et al (1995) Effects of human renin in the vasculature of rats transgenic for human angiotensinogen. Hypertension 26(2):272–278
20. Egan BM, Lu G, Greene EL (1999) Vascular effects of non-esterified fatty acids: implications for the cardiovascular risk factor cluster. Prostaglandins Leukot Essent Fatty Acids 60(5–6):411–420
21. Ross R (1999) Atherosclerosis–an inflammatory disease. N Engl J Med 340(2):115–126
22. Salgado-Somoza A, Teijeira-Fernandez E, Fernandez AL, Gonzalez-Juanatey JR, Eiras S (2010) Proteomic analysis of epicardial and subcutaneous adipose tissue reveals differences in proteins involved in oxidative stress. Am J Physiol Heart Circ Physiol 299(1):H202–H209
23. Greenstein AS, Khavandi K, Withers SB, Sonoyama K, Clancy O, Jeziorska M et al (2009) Local inflammation and hypoxia abolish the protective anticontractile properties of perivascular fat in obese patients. Circulation 119(12):1661–1670
24. Sowers JR (1991) Is hypertension an insulin-resistant state? Metabolic changes associated with hypertension and antihypertensive therapy. Am Heart J 122(3 Pt 2):932–935
25. Cersosimo E, DeFronzo RA (2006) Insulin resistance and endothelial dysfunction: the road map to cardiovascular diseases. Diabetes Metab Res Rev 22(6):423–436
26. Schneider MP, Delles C, Fleischmann E, Schmidt BM, John S, Schmieder RE (2003) Effect of elevated triglyceride levels on endothelium-dependent vasodilation in patients with hypercholesterolemia. Am J Cardiol 91(4):482–484
27. Dzau V, Braunwald E (1991) Resolved and unresolved issues in the prevention and treatment of coronary artery disease: a workshop consensus statement. Am Heart J 121(4 Pt 1):1244–1263
28. Glorioso N, Troffa C, Filigheddu F, Dettori F, Soro A, Parpaglia PP et al (1999) Effect of the HMG-CoA reductase inhibitors on blood pressure in patients with essential hypertension and primary hypercholesterolemia. Hypertension 34(6):1281–1286
29. Golomb BA, Dimsdale JE, White HL, Ritchie JB, Criqui MH (2008) Reduction in blood pressure with statins: results from the UCSD Statin Study, a randomized trial. Arch Intern Med 168(7):721–727
30. Sever PS, Dahlof B, Poulter NR, Wedel H, Beevers G, Caulfield M et al (2003) Prevention of coronary and stroke events with atorvastatin in hypertensive patients who have average or lower-than-average cholesterol concentrations, in the anglo-scandinavian cardiac outcomes trial–lipid lowering arm (ASCOT-LLA): a multicentre randomised controlled trial. Lancet 361(9364):1149–1158
31. Juncos LI, Juncos LA, Garcia NH (2012) The antihypertensive actions of statins: modulation by salt intake. Am J Hypertens 25(11):1140–1148
32. Schlaich MP, Hering D, Sobotka P, Krum H, Lambert GW, Lambert E et al (2012) Effects of renal denervation on sympathetic activation, blood pressure, and glucose metabolism in patients with resistant hypertension. Front Physiol 3:10
33. Lambert GW, Straznicky NE, Lambert EA, Dixon JB, Schlaich MP (2010) Sympathetic nervous activation in obesity and the metabolic syndrome–causes, consequences and therapeutic implications. Pharmacol Ther 126(2):159–172
34. Velliquette RA, Ernsberger P (2003) Contrasting metabolic effects of antihypertensive agents. J Pharmacol Exp Ther 307(3):1104–1111
35. Mahfoud F, Schlaich M, Kindermann I, Ukena C, Cremers B, Brandt MC et al (2011) Effect of renal sympathetic denervation on glucose metabolism in patients with resistant hypertension: a pilot study. Circulation 123(18):1940–1946

36. Hall JE, Brands MW, Henegar JR (1999) Mechanisms of hypertension and kidney disease in obesity. Ann N Y Acad Sci 892:91–107
37. Briones AM, Cat AN, Callera GE, Yogi A, Burger D, He Y et al (2012) Adipocytes produce aldosterone through calcineurin-dependent signaling pathways: implications in diabetes mellitus-associated obesity and vascular dysfunction. Hypertension 59(5):1069–1078
38. Ehrmann DA, Liljenquist DR, Kasza K, Azziz R, Legro RS, Ghazzi MN (2006) Prevalence and predictors of the metabolic syndrome in women with polycystic ovary syndrome. J Clin Endocrinol Metab 91(1):48–53
39. Reckelhoff JF (2007) Polycystic ovary syndrome: androgens and hypertension. Hypertension 49(6):1220–1221
40. Chen MJ, Yang WS, Yang JH, Chen CL, Ho HN, Yang YS (2007) Relationship between androgen levels and blood pressure in young women with polycystic ovary syndrome. Hypertension 49(6):1442–1447
41. Hacihanefioglu B, Somunkiran A, Mahmutoglu I, Sercelik A, Toptani S, Kervancioglu E (2002) Effect of hypertension therapy with the angiotensin-converting enzyme inhibitor lisinopril on hyperandrogenism in women with polycystic ovary syndrome. Fertil Steril 77(3):526–528
42. Mancia G, De Backer G, Dominiczak A, Cifkova R, Fagard R, Germano G et al (2007) 2007 ESH-ESC practice guidelines for the management of arterial hypertension: ESH-ESC task force on the management of arterial hypertension. J Hypertens 25(9):1751–1762
43. Redon J, Cifkova R, Laurent S, Nilsson P, Narkiewicz K, Erdine S et al (2008) The metabolic syndrome in hypertension: European society of hypertension position statement. J Hypertens 26(10):1891–1900
44. Grossman E, Verdecchia P, Shamiss A, Angeli F, Reboldi G (2011) Diuretic treatment of hypertension. Diabetes Care 34(Suppl 2):S313–S319
45. Mancia G, Grassi G, Zanchetti A (2006) New-onset diabetes and antihypertensive drugs. J Hypertens 24(1):3–10
46. Mancia G, Laurent S, Agabiti-Rosei E, Ambrosioni E, Burnier M, Caulfield MJ et al (2009) Reappraisal of European guidelines on hypertension management: a European society of hypertension task force document. Blood Press 18(6):308–347
47. Destro M, Cagnoni F, Dognini GP, Galimberti V, Taietti C, Cavalleri C et al (2011) Telmisartan: just an antihypertensive agent? A literature review. Expert Opin Pharmacother 12(17):2719–2735
48. Cukierman-Yaffe T, Gerstein HC, Anderson C, Zhao F, Sleight P, Hilbrich L et al (2009) Glucose intolerance and diabetes as risk factors for cognitive impairment in people at high cardiovascular risk: results from the ONTARGET/TRANSCEND research programme. Diabetes Res Clin Pract 83(3):387–393
49. Yusuf S, Teo KK, Pogue J, Dyal L, Copland I, Schumacher H et al (2008) Telmisartan, ramipril, or both in patients at high risk for vascular events. N Engl J Med 358(15):1547–1559
50. Yusuf S, Teo K, Anderson C, Pogue J, Dyal L, Copland I et al (2008) Effects of the angiotensin-receptor blocker telmisartan on cardiovascular events in high-risk patients intolerant to angiotensin-converting enzyme inhibitors: a randomised controlled trial. Lancet 372(9644):1174–1183
51. Pool JL (1991) Effects of doxazosin on serum lipids: a review of the clinical data and molecular basis for altered lipid metabolism. Am Heart J 121(1 Pt 2):251–259
52. Yamasaki Y, Shiba Y, Sekiya M, Tsujino T, Hakui N, Kawamori R et al (1994) Selective alpha 1-adrenergic inhibition improves decrease glucose disposal in patients with essential hypertension. J Hum Hypertens 8(8):555–558
53. Haenni A, Lithell H (1999) Moxonidine improves insulin sensitivity in insulin-resistant hypertensives. J Hypertens Suppl 17(3):S29–S35

54. Sowers JR, Whaley-Connell A, Epstein M (2009) Narrative review: the emerging clinical implications of the role of aldosterone in the metabolic syndrome and resistant hypertension. Ann Intern Med 150(11):776–783
55. Bhalla RC, Toth KF, Tan E, Bhatty RA, Mathias E, Sharma RV (1996) Vascular effects of metformin. Possible mechanisms for its antihypertensive action in the spontaneously hypertensive rat. Am J Hypertens 9(6):570–576
56. Zarzuelo MJ, Jimenez R, Galindo P, Sanchez M, Nieto A, Romero M et al (2011) Antihypertensive effects of peroxisome proliferator-activated receptor-beta activation in spontaneously hypertensive rats. Hypertension 58(4):733–743
57. Alberti KG, Zimmet P, Shaw J (2006) Metabolic syndrome–a new world-wide definition. A consensus statement from the international diabetes federation. Diabet Med 23(5):469–480

Cardiac and Vascular Alterations in Resistant Hypertension

4

Enrico Agabiti Rosei, Maria Lorenza Muiesan and Damiano Rizzoni

4.1 Introduction

Resistant hypertension is defined as systolic and diastolic blood pressure that remains above goal (i.e., >140/90 mmHg in the general population of hypertensive patients and >130/80 mmHg in high-risk individuals such as patients with diabetes or chronic kidney disease), despite adherence to lifestyle measures and to pharmacological treatment with full doses of at least three antihypertensive medications, including a diuretic [1]. RH is recognized as a clinical phenotype carrying a high cardiovascular risk [1].

The risk of clinical complications including stroke, acute aortic dissection, myocardial infarction, congestive heart failure, and renal failure is higher in patients with resistant hypertension, when compared with other groups of hypertensive patients, including not only well-controlled subjects, but also false resistant and masked hypertension [2–4].

In fact, Redon et al. [5] followed 86 patients with RH, for an average period of 49 months, and was able to show that the overall incidence rate of cardiovascular events was 24.6 %; the incidence of events was related to BP values (assessed by 24-h BP monitoring) increasing progressively from 2.2 per 100 patient-years in the lowest tertile of diastolic BP, to 9.5 in the intermediate tertile, and to 13.6 in the highest tertile.

More recently Daugherty et al. [6] confirmed the high rate of incident cardiovascular events in patients with RH. In that study, among 205,750 patients with hypertension, 1.9 % developed resistant hypertension, and these resistant hypertensive patients were more often men, older, and diabetics than non-resistant

E. Agabiti Rosei (✉) · M. L. Muiesan · D. Rizzoni
Clinica Medica, Department of Clinical and Experimental Sciences, University of Brescia, c/o 2a Medicina, Spedali Civili di Brescia, 25100 Brescia, Italy
e-mail: agabiti@med.unibs.it

G. Mancia (ed.), *Resistant Hypertension*, DOI: 10.1007/978-88-470-5415-8_4,

patients. The rate of cardiovascular events was significantly higher in those with RH, as compared with those without (18.0 % versus 13.5 %, $P < 0.001$), and the hazard ratio was 1.47 [confidence interval (CI) 1.33–1.62] after adjustment for patient and clinical characteristics.

Resistant or refractory hypertension (RH) represents a subset of uncontrolled BP strongly associated with organ damage, in particular at the cardiac, renal, and vascular levels [7]. The relationship between RH and cardiovascular disease/target organ damage may be bidirectional: RH may directly cause the development and worsening of target organ damage, through the persistent elevation of blood pressure. On the other hand, the presence of cardiovascular damage may contribute to worsen the resistance to treatment, making hypertension more difficult to control [8, 9].

In patients with renal disease, microvascular disease, left ventricular hypertrophy, aortic stiffness, cerebrovascular disease, or secondary hypertension, the prevalence and incidence of RH may be clearly increased.

A number of studies have analyzed the association between RH and some aspects of target organ damage, but only few of them have focused on the presence of more than one [10].

The present review is aimed to update the currently available data on the relationship between RH and subclinical damage in the heart, microcirculation, and macrocirculation.

4.2 Cardiac Damage

Among the different features of hypertensive heart disease, left ventricular hypertrophy, left ventricular dysfunction, and left atrial enlargement have been reported in RH patients.

The most frequent abnormality described in RH is LVH, assessed by both electrocardiography and echocardiography.

Cuspidi et al. [11] have identified a total of 11 cross-sectional and longitudinal studies, including 3,325 patients attending outpatient hypertension clinics and have observed that prevalence rates of echocardiographic LVH, as assessed by updated criteria, ranged from 55 to 75 % of patients with RH, peaking to 91 % in the subgroup with concomitant electrocardiographic (ECG) LV strain (Fig. 4.1). Reduction in ECG-LVH induced by treatment showed a relevant beneficial impact on cardiovascular prognosis.

A large amount of evidence on ECG and echocardiographic findings related to RH has been provided by a number of studies conducted in Brazil by Salles et al. [12–17].

In these studies, true RH patients were identified by ambulatory BP monitoring, ruling out the presence of white-coat hypertension. In 471 RH patients, the prevalence rates of ECG (Cornell's product >240 mV*ms) and echocardiographic

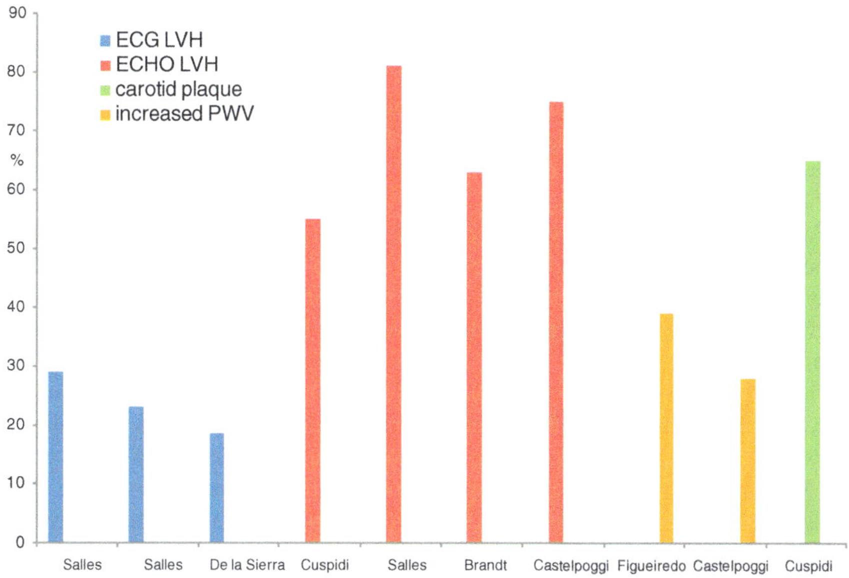

Fig. 4.1 Prevalence (%) of ECG or echocardiographic left ventricular hypertrophy (LVH), of increased aortic stiffness, and of carotid alterations in patients with RH

LVH were 29 and 81 %, respectively. Authors have initially assessed the relationship between QT interval-derived parameters and echocardiographic LVH and observed that values of QTc interval >440 ms and Cornell's product >240 mV*ms were associated respectively, with a 2.0-fold and 2.6-fold greater chance of having an increased left ventricular mass at the echocardiographic examination [12]. When the presence of a prolonged QT interval and an increased Cornell's product was combined, the relative risk of having echocardiographic LVH increased by 5.3- to 9.3-fold, compared with a normal QT interval and Cornell's product.

Salles et al. [13] have thereafter investigated the clinical significance of ECG strain pattern that was identified in 101 patients (23 %); in these patients, the prevalence rate of echocardiographic LVH was 91 %. Patients with strain were more frequently men with lower body mass index and had more target organ damage, higher 24-h blood pressure, higher serum creatinine and 24-h microalbuminuria, and more prolonged QT interval duration than those without strain. In a multivariate analysis, the presence of ECG strain was associated with increased LVM ($P < 0.001$), higher 24-h systolic blood pressure ($P < 0.001$), prolonged maximum QTc-interval duration ($P < 0.001$), lower waist circumference ($P = 0.009$), male gender ($P = 0.011$), physical inactivity ($P = 0.020$), higher serum creatinine ($P = 0.031$) and fasting glycemia ($P = 0.027$), and the presence of coronary heart disease ($P = 0.001$) and peripheral arterial disease ($P = 0.045$).

Cuspidi et al. [10] have investigated the prevalence of organ damage in the heart, carotid arteries, and kidney in 54 true RH (mean age 57 ± 10 years) and compared the findings with age- and sex-matched hypertensive patients with a good control of blood pressure using a combination of 2 or 3 drugs. LVH prevalence was higher in RH patients ranging from 40 to 55 %, in relation to the different criteria for LVH. Concentric LVH was the more common type of geometric pattern in these patients.

Castelpoggi et al. [14] have collected the largest number of RH patients with echocardiographic examination at the Rio de Janeiro University. They studied 600 patients at high or very high CV risk (23 % coronary heart disease and 15 % previous cerebrovascular events) and observed that LVH was present in 75 % of patients.

The same group of authors was able to assess the prognostic value of alterations in ECG repolarization and voltage parameters in a large group of 538 RH patients (75 % with echo LVH), prospectively followed for an average period of 4.8 years [15]. Authors have shown that among all repolarization parameters, only the QTc interval duration resulted an independent predictor of cardiovascular mortality and all-cause mortality.

In a subsequent analysis of the same database [16], the prognostic significance of serial changes on LV strain pattern (present at baseline in 21 % of RH patients) was evaluated. Persistence or development of strain during the follow-up was associated with an increased risk of stroke (hazard ratio 3.09, 95 % CI 1.40–6.81) and of death for all causes (hazard ratio 1.99, 95 % CI 1.10–3.61).

Finally, the prognostic significance of serial changes on LVH voltage criteria was analyzed in a slightly larger group of 552 patients [17]. The presence of Cornell's voltage and product criteria at baseline, but not of Sokolow-Lyon voltage, was independently associated with an increased incidence of cardiovascular morbidity and mortality and with all-cause mortality during the follow-up. In addition, the regression or the absence of ECG-LVH from baseline to follow-up was associated with a lower incidence of major cardiovascular events.

The data strongly suggest the importance of evaluating cardiac target organ damage in patients with RH, both at the initial evaluation and also during treatment [18].

Despite the fact that the evidence of the prognostic significance of LVH regression was confirmed in several studies [19, 20], only few studies have addressed the effect of antihypertensive treatment on LVH and LV mass changes in the setting of RH patients [21, 22].

De Faire et al. have compared the effects of captopril therapy (with a large dose range, from 75 to 450 mg per day) to a combination of three drugs (i.e., diuretic, beta-blocker, calcium antagonist, or direct vasodilator) in a small group of 10 patients with RH. In this study, a decrease in LV wall thickness was observed after 12 months of treatment, despite no significant changes in LV mass were shown [21].

More recently, Gaddam et al. have assessed the effects of spironolactone (25–50 mg per day) on LV mass, right ventricular, and LV volumes, measured by magnetic resonance imaging, in 34 RH patients. After 3 months of treatment with the aldosterone antagonist, a significant decrease in LV mass, in LV wall thickness and volume, and in left atrial size was observed, and the effect was greater in the group of 19 patients with RH due to primary aldosteronism [23].

The effect of renal denervation on echocardiographic LV mass has been demonstrated by Brandt et al. in 46 RH patients, compared with 18 controls receiving only medical treatment (mean number of drugs 4.7) [24]. At echocardiographic controls performed 1 and 6 months from baseline, LVM and the E/E′ ratio (index of increased LV filling pressure) were significantly reduced after the renal denervation procedure, while these did not change during medical treatment. In the whole group of patients, the improvement in LV mass index and E/E′ ratio was related to the decrease in BP induced by treatment, although it was observed also in those patients defined as "non-responders" on the basis of clinic BP values, suggesting some additional effect of sympathetic renal denervation of cardiac target organ damage, independent of pressure load.

4.3 Large Arteries

A relation exists between vascular calcification, arterial stiffness, and difficult to control hypertension. In patients with RH, the presence of structural alterations in large caliber vessels, such as carotid arteries and aorta, may have a great impact of blood pressure control [25].

In some studies, an increased prevalence of carotid wall thickness, atherosclerotic plaques, and aortic stiffness has been demonstrated.

Cuspidi et al. [10] for the first time documented the increased prevalence of intima-media thickening or of plaques in the carotid arteries of RH patients as compared with a group of patients treated with a combination of antihypertensive drugs, but with controlled BP values in the clinic and during 24-h BP monitoring (prevalence 58 and 65 % versus 29 and 32 %, respectively).

It was also suggested that among patients with carotid arteries stenosis, the prevalence of RH was fairly high. Spence et al. analyzed 170 patients with carotid arteries stenosis who participated in the North American Symptomatic Carotid Endarterectomy Trial or the Asymptomatic Carotid Artery Study and observed that RH was present in 79 (47 %) related to renovascular hypertension in 20 and to adrenocortical hyperplasia in 7 [26].

More recently, Schmieder et al. analyzed the presence of vascular target organ damage in 42 RH patients, who were investigated by brain magnetic resonance imaging. Twenty-three patients had cerebral microangiopathy that was associated with higher systolic blood pressure during nighttime. In addition, RH patients with cerebral microangiopathy had similar carotid intima-media thickness but higher pulse wave velocity, central pulse pressure, and aortic augmentation pressure [27].

Some other studies have evaluated the increase in aortic stiffness in patients with RH. Figueiredo et al. have measured carotid femoral pulse wave velocity in 44 patients with RH, 35 patients with controlled blood pressure values, and 25 normotensive subjects, showing a significant increase in PWV in patients with RH as compared with the other 2 groups [28]. Since endothelial function may contribute to the regulation of large artery elasticity, authors have also evaluated flow-mediated changes in the vessel diameter and observed that a greater decrease in brachial artery flow-mediated vasodilation was more evident in RH when compared with well-controlled hypertensive patients.

In the largest cross-sectional study including 600 resistant hypertensive patients without peripheral arterial disease, Castelpoggi et al. [14] assessed arterial stiffness by aortic pulse wave velocity (PWV) measurements and found that 168 patients (28 %) had aortic PWV >12 m/s. Patients with increased PWV were older and had a higher prevalence of cardiovascular risk factors than did those patients with normal PWV. A blunted nocturnal decrease in BP was independently associated with increased aortic stiffness in RH patients, together with older age, diabetes, microalbuminuria, low HDL cholesterol, and a widened 24-h BP.

4.4 Microcirculation

In hypertension, small artery remodeling is the most prevalent form and one of the first manifestations of target organ damage. The magnitude of remodeling of small resistance arteries in hypertension has been demonstrated to have prognostic significance with worse prognosis for subjects with greater structural alterations, as evaluated by the media thickness/lumen diameter ratio [29].

The available evidence shows that in patients with secondary hypertension (and a greater prevalence of RH), the increase in the media-to-lumen ratio is particularly pronounced in comparison with essential hypertensive patients [30]. Most interestingly in patients with renovascular hypertension and to a lesser extent in those with primary aldosteronism, a more evident contribution of cell growth, leading to the development of hypertrophic remodeling, (indicating smooth muscle cell growth), has been observed. In addition, a more pronounced fibrosis in the tunica media, in terms of total collagen content, with a more evident increase in collagen type III, has been demonstrated in patients with primary aldosteronism [31] (Fig. 4.2). In the development of hypertrophic remodeling, a relevant role is played by growth factors, especially endothelin-1 and angiotensin II, while the mechanisms leading to eutrophic remodeling (increased media-to-lumen ratio without muscle cell growth) are less clear. Endothelin-1 is a powerful vasoconstrictor and mitogen, contributing to the elevation of blood pressure and related target organ damage. Vascular effects of aldosterone may be mediated, as suggested by Schiffrin et al., by the stimulation of endothelin production. In patients with RH, the content of endothelin -1 was significantly greater than in mild hypertensive patients or normotensive controls [32].

The evaluation of retinal vessels may represent a method for the evaluation of microcirculation. Cuspidi et al. [10] observed that patients with RH, undergoing a traditional fundoscopic examination, had a very high rate of retinal vascular

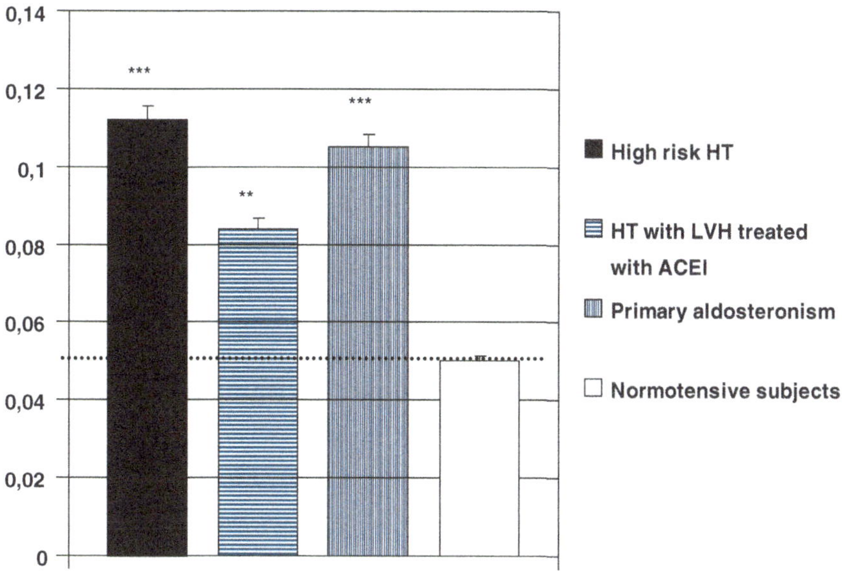

Fig. 4.2 Media thickness/lumen diameter ratio (M/L) in patients at high cardiovascular risk, in patents with primary aldosteronism, in patients with essential hypertension, and in normotensive subjects

changes (narrowings and arteriovenous crossings) and a greater prevalence of grade 2 and 3 retinopathy (73 and 5 %), according to the Keith–Wagener classification, as compared with a control group (38 and 0 %).

Another study examined the fundus oculi in 497 patients, of whom 63 % with true RH and 37 % with white-coat hypertension, and the results confirmed a higher prevalence of retinopathy in true resistant patients (55.2 vs. 40 %, P = 0.002) [33].

More recently, measurements of retinal arterioles have been taken in vivo with scanning laser doppler flowmetry in 40 patients with resistant hypertension. All the parameters indicating the presence of microvascular abnormalities, that is, the wall-to-lumen ratio, the wall thickness, and the wall cross section area, were strongly associated with urinary sodium excretion and less consistently with 24-h blood pressure. In this group of patients, urinary sodium excretion represented the only independent determinant of wall thickness and of wall cross section area of retinal arterioles. Since retinal arteriolar alterations are related to cerebral vascular structure, these results might prove to have important implications on risk stratification in patients with resistant hypertension [34].

We have investigated the possible predictive effect of vascular structural alterations in relation to the time course of blood pressure after surgical correction of primary aldosteronism [35]. We calculated receiver-operating characteristic curves for identification of patients with aldosterone-producing adenoma, who achieved normotension post-adrenalectomy, compared with those who did not [35]. For both the media-to-lumen ratio of subcutaneous small arteries, evaluated before surgical correction, and known duration of hypertension, the area under the curve differed significantly from the area under the curve under the identity line, thus indicating the usefulness of either variable for predicting the outcome on blood pressure in these patients [35]. Therefore, the extent of alterations of microcirculation predicts the pressor outcome after adrenalectomy, both in terms of absolute blood pressure values and/or in terms of number or doses of drugs needed.

4.5 Concomitant Cardiac and Vascular Damage

Few studies have evaluated the association between RH and the presence of more than one target organ damage [10, 14, 27] and have found a correlation between cardiac, vascular, and renal damage in patients with resistant hypertension.

In the Vobarno Study, the prevalence of resistant hypertension and the presence and degree of associated cardiac, vascular, and renal target organ damage were assessed in a general population sample, participating in a prospective epidemiological study, originally aimed to measure the association between cardiovascular risk factors and target organ damage (Vobarno Study) [36, 37]. Resistant hypertension prevalence was 9,5 % according to the definition proposed by Calhoun et al. [1], and in RH individuals, a higher LV mass index, PWV, and carotid intima-media thickness are shown (Figs. 4.3, 4.4 and 4.5) [38], confirming and extending previous results.

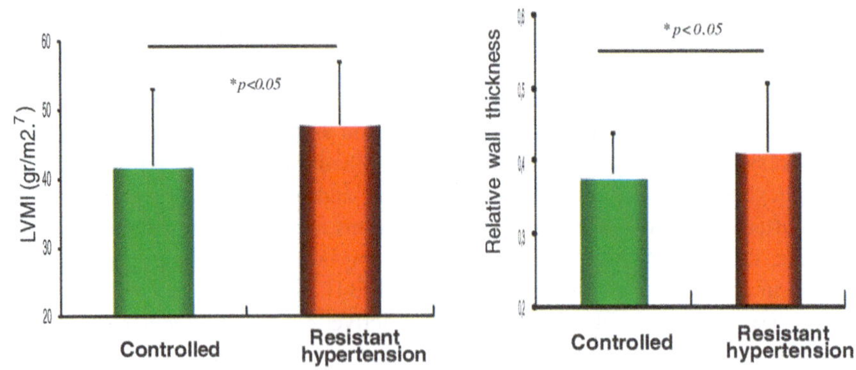

Fig. 4.3 Left ventricular mass index in resistant and controlled hypertensives

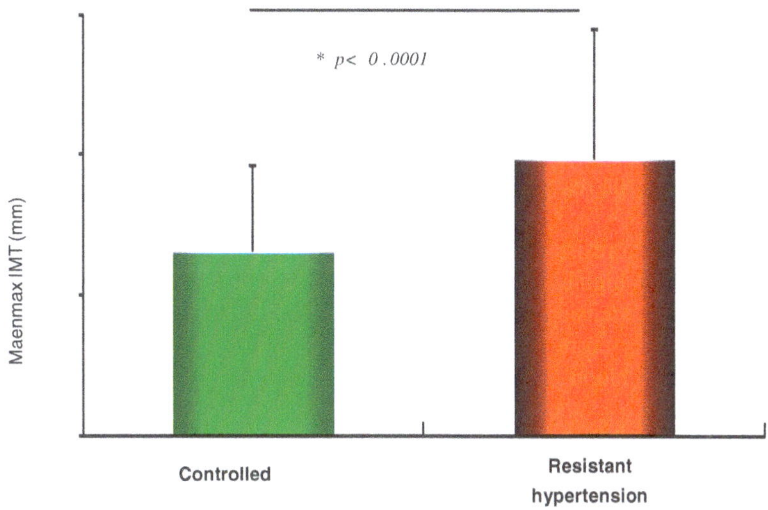

Fig. 4.4 Intima-media thickness in resistant and controlled hypertensives

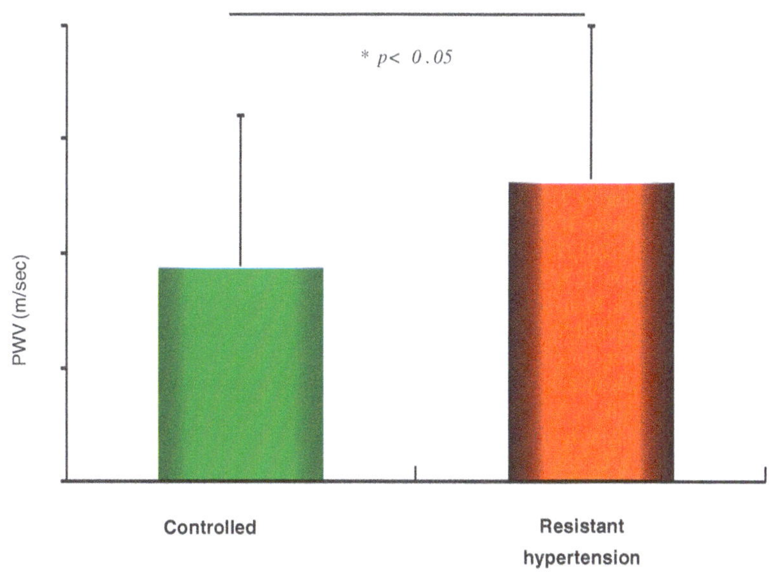

Fig. 4.5 Pulse wave velocity in resistant and controlled hypertensives

4.6 Conclusions

- Resistant hypertension is associated with multiple cardiovascular risk factors and organ damage.
- The proportion of patients with clinical target organ damage is greater in subjects with true resistant hypertension than in those with white-coat resistant hypertension.
- In patients with resistant hypertension, subclinical organ damage itself may be responsible for high blood pressure values, but it is also the result of detrimental effects of hypertension on large arteries as well as on the microvascular network. The early correction of such vascular abnormalities is vital for medium- and long-term blood pressure control.

References

1. Calhoun D 1. A, Jones D, Textor S, Goff DC, Murphy TP, Toto RD, et al. (2008) Resistant hypertension: diagnosis, evaluation, and treatment. A scientific statement from the American Heart Association Professional Education Committee of the Council for High Blood Pressure Research. Circulation 117:e510–e526
2. Hall WD (2002) Resistant hypertension, secondary hypertension, and hypertensive crises. Cardiol Clin 20:281–289
3. Pierdomenico SD, Lapenna D, Bucci A, Di Tommaso R, Di Mascio R, Manente BM et al (2005) Cardiovascular outcome in treated hypertensive patients with responder, masked, false resistant, and true resistant hypertension. Am J Hypertens 18:1422–1428
4. Papadopoulos DP, Papademetriou V (2006) Resistant hypertension: diagnosis and management. J Cardiovasc Pharmacol Ther 11:113–118
5. Redon J, Campos C, Narciso ML, Rodicio JL, Pascual JM, Ruilope LM (1998) Prognostic value of ambulatory blood pressure monitoring in refractory hypertension. A prospective study. Hypertension 31:712–718
6. Daugherty SL, Powers JD, Magid DJ, Tavel HM, Masoudi FA, Margolis KL, O'Connor PJ, Selby JV, Ho PM (2012) Incidence and prognosis of resistant hypertension in hypertensive patients. Circulation 125:1635–1642
7. Guidelines for the Management of Arterial Hypertension (2007) The task force for the management of arterial hypertension of the European society of hypertension (ESH) and of the European society of cardiology (ESC). J Hypertens 25:1105–1187
8. McAlister FA, Lewanczuk RZ, Teo KK (1996) Resistant hypertension: an overview. Can J Cardiol 12:822–828
9. Ram CVS (2003) Management of refractory hypertension. Am J Therapeut 10:122–126
10. Cuspidi C, Macca G, Sampieri L, Michev I, Salerno M, Fusi V, Severgnini B, Meani S, Magrini F, Zanchetti A (2001) High prevalence of cardiac and extracardiac target organ damage in refractory hypertension. J Hypertens 19(11):2063–2070
11. Cuspidi C, Vaccarella A, Negri F, Sala C (2010) Resistant hypertension and left ventricular hypertrophy: an overview. J Am Soc Hypertens 4(6):319–324
12. Salles G, Leocadio S, Bloch K, Nogueira AR, Muxfeldt E (2005) Combined QT interval and voltage criteria improve left ventricular hypertrophy detection in resistant hypertension. Hypertension 46:1207–1212
13. Salles G, Cardoso C, Nogueira AR, Bloch K, Muxfeldt E (2006) Importance of the electrocardiographic strain pattern in patients with resistant hypertension. Hypertension 48:437–442

14. Castelpoggi CH, Pereira VS, Fiszman R, Cardoso CRL, Muxfeldt ES, Salles G (2009) A blunted decrease in nocturnal blood pressure is independently associated with increased aortic stiffness in patients with resistant hypertension. Hypertens Res 32:591–596
15. Salles G, Cardoso CRL, Muxfeldt E (2009) Prognostic value of ventricular repolarization prolongation in resistant hypertension: a prospective cohort study. J Hypertens 27:1094–1101
16. Salles G, Cardoso CRL, Fiszman R, Muxfeldt ES (2010) Prognostic significance of baseline and serial changes in electrocardiographic strain pattern in resistant hypertension. J Hypertens 28:1715–1733
17. Salles G, Cardoso CRL, Fiszman R, Muxfeldt ES (2010) Prognostic impact of baseline and serial changes in electrocardiographic left ventricular hypertrophy in resistant hypertension. Am Heart J 159:833–840
18. Hernandez-del Rey R, Armario P, Martin-Baranera M, Sanchez P, Cardenas G, Pardell H (1998) Target-organ damage and cardiovascular risk profile in resistant hypertension. Influence of the white-coat effect. Blood Press Monit 3:331–337
19. Armstrong AC, Gidding S, Gjesdal O, Wu C, Bluemke DA, Lima JA (2012) LV mass assessed by echocardiography and CMR, cardiovascular outcomes, and medical practice. JACC Cardiovasc Imaging 5(8):837–848
20. Muiesan ML, Salvetti M, Rizzoni D, Castellano M, Donato F, Agabiti-Rosei E (1995) Association of change in left ventricular mass with prognosis during long-term antihypertensive treatment. J Hypertens 13(10):1091–1095
21. de Faire U, Lindwall K, Andersson G, Eriksson S (1989) Regression of left ventricular hypertrophy on long-term treatment with captopril of severe hypertensives refractory to standard triple treatment. Eur J Clin Pharmacol 37:291–294
22. Julien J, Dufloux MA, Prasquier R, Chatellier G, Menard D, Plouin PF et al (1990) Effects of captopril and minoxidil on left ventricular hypertrophy in resistant hypertensive patients: a 6 month double-blind comparison. J Am Coll Cardiol 16:137–142
23. Gaddam K, Corros C, Pimenta E, Ahmed M, Denney T, Aban I et al (2010) Rapid reversal of left ventricular hypertrophy and intracardiac volume in patients with resistant hypertension and hyperaldosteronism. A prospective clinical study. Hypertension 55:1137–1142
24. Brandt MC, Mahfoud F, Reda S, Schirmer SH, Erdmann E, Böhm M, Hoppe UC (2012) Renal sympathetic denervation reduces left ventricular hypertrophy and improves cardiac function in patients with resistant hypertension. J Am Coll Cardiol 59:901–909
25. Pickering TG (2007) Arterial stiffness as a cause of resistant hypertension? J Clin Hypertens 9:390–395
26. Spence JD (2000) Management of resistant hypertension in patients with carotid stenosis: high prevalence of renovascular hypertension. Cerebrovasc Dis 10(4):249–254
27. Schmieder RE, Schmidt BM, Raff U, Bramlage P, Dörfler A, Achenbach S, Schwab J, Kolominsky-Rabas P (2011) Cerebral microangiopathy in treatment-resistant hypertension. Clin Hypertens 13(8):582–587
28. Figueiredo VN, Yugar-Toledo JC, Martins LC, Martins LB, de Faria AP, de Haro Moraes C, Sierra C, Coca A, Moreno H (2012) Vascular stiffness and endothelial dysfunction: correlations at different levels of blood pressure. Blood Press 21(1):31–38
29. Rizzoni D, Porteri E, Boari GE et al (2003) Prognostic significance of small-artery structure in hypertension. Circulation 108:2230–2235
30. Rizzoni D, Porteri E, Castellano M, Bettoni G, Muiesan ML, Muiesan P, Giulini SM, Agabiti Rosei E (1996) Vascular hypertrophy and remodeling in secondary hypertension. Hypertension 28:785–790
31. Rizzoni D, Paiardi S, Rodella L, Porteri E, De Ciuceis C, Rezzani R, Boari GE, Zani F, Miclini M, Tiberio GA, Giulini SM, Rosei CA, Bianchi R, Agabiti Rosei E (2006) Changes in extracellular matrix in subcutaneous small resistance arteries of patients with primary aldosteronism. J Clin Endocrinol Metab 91(7):2638–2642
32. Schiffrin EL, Deng LY, Sventek P, Day R (1997) Enhanced expression of endothelin-1 gene in resistance arteries in severe human essential hypertension. J Hypertens 15(1):57–63

33. Muxfeldt ES, Bloch KV, Nogueira Ada R, Salles GF (2005) True resistant hypertension: is it possible to be recognized in the office? Am J Hypertens 18:1534–1540
34. Raff U, Harazny JM, Titze SI, Schmidt BM, Michelson G, Schmieder RE (2012) Salt intake determines retinal arteriolar structure in treatment resistant hypertension independent of blood pressure. Atherosclerosis 222(1):235–240
35. Rossi GP, Bolognesi M, Rizzoni D, Seccia TM, Piva A, Porteri E, Tiberio GA, Giulini SM, Agabiti-Rosei E, Pessina AC (2008) Vascular remodeling and duration of hypertension predict outcome of adrenalectomy in primary aldosteronism patients. Hypertension 51(5):1366–1371
36. Muiesan ML, Salvetti M, Zulli R, Pasini GF, Bettoni G, Monteduro C et al (1998) Structural association between the carotid artery and the left ventricle in a general population in Northern Italy: the Vobarno study. J Hypertens 16(Pt 1):1805–1812
37. Muiesan ML, Salvetti M, Paini A, Monteduro C, Rosei CA, Aggiusti C, Belotti E, Bertacchini F, Galbassini G, Stassaldi D, Castellano M, Rosei EA (2010) Pulse wave velocity and cardiovascular risk stratification in a general population: the Vobarno study. J Hypertens 28:1935–1943
38. Salvetti M, Muiesan ML, Paini A, Agabiti Rosei C, Aggiusti C, Bertacchini F, Stassaldi D, Beschi F, Cobelli S, Rubagotti G, Monteduro C, Castellano M, Agabiti Rosei E (2011) Resistant hypertension in a general population in Northern Italy: prevalence, associated cardiovascular risk factors and target organ damage. J Hypertens 29 (suppl A) 42.362. (abst)

5 The Pathophysiology of the Kidney in Resistant Hypertension

Hermann Haller

The kidney plays a major role in the regulation of blood pressure and the pathogenesis of hypertension [1–3]. In particular in a state of resistant hypertension, that is, massively increased blood pressure which is resistant to antihypertensive medication, it is important to understand how the kidney influences blood pressure in order to define its contribution to the "resistant state" and to delineate a mechanism-based therapeutic strategy.

The dominant role of the kidney for blood pressure regulation is due to the fact that the kidney is implicated on several levels in the maintenance of blood pressure and its pathological elevation. The kidney has three levels on which it influences blood pressure. Firstly, the kidney is the major organ to regulate blood volume via the retention (or excretion) of salt and water. Secondly, the kidney influences vascular tone by release of vasoactive hormones such as renin. Last but not least, the kidney contributes to the activity of the sympathetic nervous system via renal afferent nerves. In resistant hypertension, the kidney may contribute on all three levels in the pathological increase in blood pressure. It is therefore important in an individual patient with resistant hypertension to assess the different renal mechanisms and their contribution to hypertension, its physiology in blood pressure regulation, and the pathophysiological implications of renal disease contributing to resistant hypertension.

Furthermore, of all blood pressure regulating systems such as the central nervous system, the heart, and the blood vessels, it is mostly the kidneys which have the ability of long-term adjustments in blood pressure [4]. This long-term adjustment of blood pressure is predominantly through the regulation of extracellular volume. In addition, the sympathetic renal outflow of the kidneys and the

H. Haller (✉)
Hannover Medical School, Clinic of Hypertension and Nephrology,
Carl-Neuberg-Strasse 1, 30625 Hannover, Germany
e-mail: Haller.hermann@mh-hannover.de

G. Mancia (ed.), *Resistant Hypertension*, DOI: 10.1007/978-88-470-5415-8_5,

secretion of vasoactive hormones may contribute to the development of a form of hypertension which is mostly resistant to treatment.

To fully understand the role of the kidney in complicated forms of hypertension, it is also important to understand that damage to the kidneys or diseased kidneys very often leads to an increase in blood pressure. In fact, high blood pressure is one of the hallmarks of renal disease. Also in the diseased kidney, the above-described three fundamental mechanisms are active: increased release of vasoactive hormones, elevated neuronal output, and enhanced retention of salt and water. In the diagnostic workup of hypertensive patients with suspected secondary forms of hypertension, the kidney is the predominant culprit. And very high blood pressure can often be attributed to the kidney. Renal vascular and renal parenchymal forms of hypertension are responsible for high blood pressure in about 10 % of hypertensive patient. In most epidemiological studies, 50 % of the renal origin of hypertension is renovascular. Renovascular or renal parenchymal hypertension is mostly recognized by high, sustained blood pressure. Since severe or refractory hypertension is the hallmark of resistant hypertension, the percentage of kidney disease in patients with resistant hypertension is more likely higher than in patients with treatable forms of hypertension. In addition, it has been suggested that also in patients with so-called essential hypertension, structural and functional alterations of the kidney contribute to the increase in blood pressure. Figure 5.1 gives an overview on the pathophysiological mechanisms in both renovascular and renal parenchymal diseases of the kidney.

5.1 Renoparenchymal Hypertension

The term renoparenchymal hypertension includes a variety of renal diseases which are characterized by either glomerular or interstitial renal disease. Clinically one can distinguish at two different conditions, that is, acute and chronic, in the renal parenchyma which is associated with hypertension. As shown in Fig. 5.1, all mechanisms which lead to tubulointerstitial disease in the kidney may lead to an increase in blood pressure and hypertension. However, clinically one can distinguish more acute and severe diseases of the kidney such as vasculitis and glomerulonephritis, which lead not only to high blood pressure but also to damage to the kidney which is diagnosed by renal function and/or urine analysis. In contrast, most hypertensive patients may have insidious parenchymal alterations in the kidney. The effects of non-steroidal drugs, resistant hypertension over a period of time, overactivity of the sympathetic nervous system, aging, and other causes may lead first to microvascular damage, followed by nephron loss and to a reduction in nephron number [4]. This tubulointerstitial disease in the kidney is clinically not associated with the loss of renal function for a long time and may only show mild forms of albuminuria, the so-called microalbuminuria. Nonetheless, these more subtle changes in the renal parenchyma may aggravate blood pressure and participate in resistant hypertension. The mechanism whereby renal parenchymal

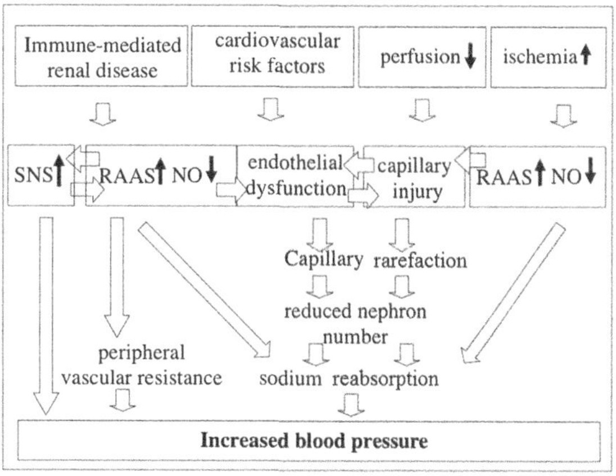

Fig. 5.1 Schema of renal pathophysiology in resistant hypertension leading from acute and/or chronic injury to interstitial disease and subsequent activation of blood pressure raising mechanisms

disease influences blood pressure is complex and only partially understood. Risk factors such as hypertension, hypercholesterolemia, and very often diabetes mellitus lead to a damage in the interstitial blood vessels in the kidney. Endothelial cell dysfunction followed by underperfusion of the renal microcirculation leads to verification of blood vessels, followed by the loss of tubules and nephrons. Since the kidney is equipped with more than 1 million nephrons, for a long time, the loss of nephrons does not lead to renal insufficiency but results in adaptive mechanisms in the kidney. A loss of nephrons leads to increased perfusion in the remaining nephrons, followed by an increase in glomerular pressure. Concomitantly, there is an increase in tubular sodium reabsorption, leading to an increased plasma volume. This volume overload although subtle and not clinically recognizable plays an important part in the development of blood pressure and may contribute to severe and resistant hypertension.

A second mechanism in renoparenchymal hypertension whereby the loss of microvasculature and nephrons may contribute to the development of resistant hypertension is an increased activity of the sympathetic nervous system. The hypoperfused microcirculation leads to an activation of efferent renal nerves. These sympathetic nerves influence the central nervous system and increase blood pressure. A third important mechanism is the release of vasoactive hormones such as renin from the hypoperfused kidneys. In order to restore renal blood flow, the release of renin is enhanced. Although increased circulating levels of angiotensin II cannot be measured in most patients, the intrarenal activity of the renin–angiotensin system is increased, contributing to sodium reabsorption, vasoconstriction, and activation of sympathetic renal nerves [5–7].

It is obvious that these insidious renal parenchymal changes may contribute to the increased blood pressure in patients with severe and refractory hypertension. Since at least three different pathophysiological mechanisms are implicated in these forms of hypertension, antihypertensive medication should be directed at all three of these pathophysiological mechanisms.

In addition to these more insidious changes in the kidney (which are more common), active renal parenchymal disease such as glomerulonephritis and/or vasculitis leads also to an increase in blood pressure. The above-described mechanisms are all activated in patients with inflammatory renal disease. The extent of the neurohumoral activation is much more severe and is accompanied by edema formation and hypertensive crisis. However, more subtle clinical forms of these diseases may not be easily recognized in the clinic and have to be diagnosed by urine analysis and renal biopsy.

On renal biopsy, the early forms of renal interstitial disease are difficult to demonstrate. Often, there is evidence of glomerular and tubulointerstitial ischemias with shrinkage of the glomerular tuft, tubular atrophy, and interstitial fibrosis. In a minority of patients, there is evidence of glomerulosclerosis in severe tubulointerstitial injury. These biopsies are termed nephrosclerosis. In cases with more severe hypertension, the artery lesion is more of a proliferative arteriolopathy sometimes with fibrinoid necrosis. Rarely, the well-described concentric layers of connected tissue and cells may give an onion-skin appearance to the vessels. In the more severe forms of renal disease, the distinct forms of acute glomerulonephritis can be observed on renal biopsy. The classical glomerulonephritis with high blood pressure is focal–segmental glomerulosclerosis.

Most patients with resistant hypertension will have a relatively normal or slightly depressed glomerular filtration rate. However, renal blood flow will be reduced, and elevated renal vascular resistance can be measured by duplex ultrasound. As described above, despite the relatively normal renal function, renal biopsy usually shows arteriosclerosis and hyalinosis in the afferent arterial and interlobular arteries.

In less than 50 % of the patients, there will be microalbuminuria, and only in a minority of patients, proteinuria will further develop.

5.2 Renal Vascular Hypertension

Renovascular hypertension is the most common form of secondary hypertension. A renal artery stenosis may clinically be diagnosed by severe refractory hypertensive crisis. Acutely increased blood pressure resistant to antihypertensive treatment is one of the hallmarks of the most common form of secondary hypertension, that is, renal artery stenosis. In all patients with resistant hypertension, renal artery stenosis as well as renal parenchymal disease has to be ruled out. However, the diagnosis of a functionally relevant renal artery stenosis in patients with resistant hypertension is not easy.

Renovascular disease may be described as two pathophysiological entities, as suggested by Textor [8, 9]. In the early stages of a functional renal artery stenosis, impaired blood flow with reactive release of vasoactive substances is predominant. In chronic stages of renal artery stenosis, ischemia is the main feature of the disease. Hypertension develops in patients with renovascular disease from a complex set of pressor signals, including activation of the renin–angiotensin system, recruitment of oxidative stress pathways, and sympathoadrenergic activation. Although the kidney maintains function over a broad range of autoregulation, sustained reduction in renal perfusion leads to disturbed microvascular function, vascular rarefaction, and ultimately development of interstitial fibrosis. The functional consequence of an acute stenosis in the larger renal blood vessels is impaired renal blood supply and ischemia. The most common form of renovascular hypertension is unilateral or bilateral atherosclerosis of the renal artery. In contrast, fibromuscular disease of the renal artery is less common and mostly prevalent in young females. Rare causes of renovascular hypertension are renal artery aneurysm, arterial embolism, or arteriovenous fistula.

It is important to understand that the presence of a vascular stenotic lesion as seen in duplex ultrasound or by angiography is not enough to establish its role for an increase in arterial pressure and leading to high, resistant hypertension. Most studies have shown that the cross-sectional area of the renal artery has to be less than 30–20 % before functional consequences develop [10]. Once the critical level is reached, several intrarenal mechanisms may occur. A central mechanism is the release of renin from the juxtaglomerular apparatus, leading to activation of the renin–angiotensin–aldosterone system with an increase in renal artery resistance and increased sodium in water reabsorption. The activation of these mechanisms can occur without the loss of renal size or function. However, over time, the renovascular impairment leads to chronic ischemia in the kidney. The local ischemia in the kidney contributes via activation of the renin–angiotensin–system but also via activation of renal sympathetic nerve activity to the maintenance and persistence of high blood pressure [11–13]. It seems obvious that in long-standing renal arteries stenosis, the intrarenal mechanisms may come independent and renal ischemia may contribute via parenchymal changes to the high, resistant blood pressure.

5.3 Conclusion

The kidney plays an important role in the development of resistant hypertension. Historically, the renal pathophysiology in hypertension has been divided into renovascular and renoparenchymal changes. If a severe renovascular stenosis is present or, on the other hand, active inflammatory disease in the renal parenchymal is present, such a diagnosis is justified. More often, the kidney is involved in resistant hypertension in a more subtle manner. Several pathological mechanisms may lead to either functional deterioration of the kidney with regional ischemia or the loss of nephrons. The pathological factors that contribute to these events range from cardiovascular risk factors such as hypertension itself, hypercholesterolemia, and/or diabetes mellitus to the intake of damaging drugs such as non-steroidal. Acute renal disease such as glomerulonephritis and/or vasculitis also leads to activation of neurohormonal axis and vascular injury. The result of the acute or chronic damage to the kidney factors is tubulointerstitial injury either directly to the tubules or, more often, via injury to the microcirculation, especially the endothelial cells. Eventually, rarefaction of the renal microcirculation will lead to ischemia with the subsequent loss of nephrons. Hyperperfusion of the remaining nephrons leads to increased glomerular pressure with subsequent loss of these remaining nephrons. Interstitial renal disease leads to (a) increased reabsorption of sodium and water, (b) increased sympathetic activity in the kidney, and (c) increased activation of the renin–angiotensin–aldosterone system. All three renal mechanisms contribute in their respective ways to the maintenance of blood pressure and may contribute to the clinical syndrome of resistant hypertension.

References

1. Wadei HM, Textor SC (2012) The role of the kidney in regulating arterial blood pressure. Nat Rev Nephrol 8(10):602–609
2. Shimosawa T, Mu S, Shibata S, Fujita T (2012) The kidney and hypertension: pathogenesis of salt-sensitive hypertension. Curr Hypertens Rep 14(5):468–472
3. Chen D, Coffman TM (2012) The kidney and hypertension: lessons from mouse models. Can J Cardiol 28(3):305–310
4. Helal I, Fick-Brosnahan GM, Reed-Gitomer B, Schrier RW (2012) Glomerular hyper filtration: definitions, mechanisms and clinical implications. Nat Rev Nephrol 8(5):293–300
5. Johnson RJ, Herrera-Acosta J, Schreiner GF, Rodriguez-Iturbe B (2002) Subtle acquired renal injury as a mechanism of salt-sensitive hypertension. N Engl J Med 346(12):913–923
6. Calhoun DA (2013) Hyperaldosteronism as a common cause of resistant hypertension. Annu Rev Med 64:233–247
7. Parati G, Esler M (2012) The human sympathetic nervous system: its relevance in hypertension and heart failure. Eur Heart J 33(9):1058–1066
8. Zanoli L, Rastelli S, Marcantoni C, Tamburino C, Laurent S, Boutouyrie P, Castellino P (2012) Renal artery diameter, renal function and resistant hypertension in patients with low-to-moderate renal artery stenosis. J Hypertens 30(3):600–607
9. Textor SC, Lerman L (2010) Renovascular hypertension and ischemic nephropathy. Am J Hypertens 23(11):1159–1169
10. Raff U, Schmidt BM, Schwab J, Schwarz TK, Achenbach S, Bär I, Schmieder RE (2010) Renal resistive index in addition to low-grade albuminuria complements screening for target organ damage in therapy-resistant hypertension. J Hypertens 28(3):608–614
11. Agarwal R (2010) Relative plasma volume monitoring for identifying volume-sensitive and resistant hypertension. Semin Dial 23(5):462–465
12. DiBona GF (2002) Sympathetic nervous system and the kidney in hypertension. Curr Opin Nephrol Hypertens 11(2):197–200
13. DiBona GF (2000) Nervous kidney, Interaction between renal sympathetic nerves and the renin-angiotensin system in the control of renal function. Hypertension 36(6):1083–1088

Part II
Diagnostic Aspects

False Versus True Resistant Hypertension

6

Gianfranco Parati, Juan E. Ochoa and Grzegorz Bilo

6.1 Introduction

While in interventional studies and in clinical practice much attention has been given to the issues related to the treatment of resistant hypertension, only marginal attention has been devoted to the methodological aspects related to BP measurement that should be considered for a proper identification of resistant hypertension. Current definition of resistant hypertension (i.e., failure to control BP by a treatment based on adequate doses of a diuretic and two additional antihypertensive drugs) is still based on office blood pressure (BP) measurements obtained in the medical office, which are characterized by important acknowledged limitations among which the frequent interference by the "white-coat" effect. Following the introduction of ABPM and HBPM in clinical practice, several studies have repeatedly reported substantial disagreements between in-office and out-of-office BP measurement techniques, leading to identification of two new forms of hypertension, previously unknown when BP measurements were limited to the clinical setting: (1) the so-called white-coat hypertension (elevated in-office but normal out-of-office BP levels) and (2) "masked" hypertension (normal in-office

G. Parati (✉) · J. E. Ochoa
Department of Health Sciences, and Department of Cardiology,
University of Milano-Bicocca and S. Luca Hospital,
IRCCS Istituto Auxologico Italiano, P.zza Brescia, 20, 20149 Milan, Italy
e-mail: gianfranco.parati@unimib.it

J. E. Ochoa
e-mail: juaneugenioo@gmail.com

G. Bilo
Department of Cardiology, S. Luca Hospital, IRCCS Istituto Auxologico Italiano,
P.zza Brescia, 20, 20149 Milan, Italy
e-mail: g.bilo@auxologico.it

G. Mancia (ed.), *Resistant Hypertension*, DOI: 10.1007/978-88-470-5415-8_6,

but elevated out-of-office BP levels) [1, 2]. Although these terms were initially defined referring to subjects not yet receiving antihypertensive treatment during the initial diagnostic approach of hypertension, equivalent phenomena have been described among treated hypertensive subjects and are known as false resistant/uncontrolled hypertension (white-coat resistant/uncontrolled hypertension, WCRH) and false BP control (masked resistant/uncontrolled hypertension (masked resistant/uncontrolled hypertension, MRH). Remarkably, observational and interventional studies implementing both in-office and out-of-office BP measurements for assessment of BP control have shown a substantial and sometimes higher-than-expected frequency of WCRH and MRH among treated hypertensive patients [3–5], indicating that OBP alone is insufficient to reliably assess BP control. Detection of these conditions with out-of-office BP monitoring is thus an essential step in the diagnostic approach to resistant hypertension. While identification of WCRH may avoid performing unnecessary and costly diagnostic tests, or exposing subjects to the adverse effects associated with multidrug therapy, detection of MRH would allow early implementation of adequate BP-lowering strategies to achieve daily-life BP control, thus preventing the adverse cardiovascular consequences associated with this condition. The present chapter is aimed at addressing the initial diagnostic approach to the patient who presents with resistant hypertension in the medical office focusing on the role of ABPM and HBPM in defining whether the failure to achieve OBP control actually corresponds to true resistant hypertension. A general outlook to the advantages of implementing out-of-office BP measuring techniques for assessment of BP control in treated hypertensive patients is also provided.

6.2 True and False Resistant Hypertension (White-Coat Resistant Hypertension): Definitions and Contributing Factors

Although different definitions have been proposed, a recent scientific statement from the American Heart Association Professional Education Committee of the Council for High Blood Pressure Research defined resistant hypertension as the persistence of BP values that remain above the OBP goal (i.e., $\geq$140/90 mmHg for diastolic/systolic BP; or $\geq$130/80 mmHg for patients with diabetes mellitus, renal dysfunction, or at high/very high CV risk) despite the concomitant use of 3 optimally dosed antihypertensive medications from different classes at near-maximal US Food and Drug Administration–approved doses, one of which should ideally be a diuretic [6]. Hypertensive patients on $\geq$4 antihypertensive drugs to achieve BP control as well as patients who have uncontrolled BP and taking 3 drugs being intolerant to diuretics are also considered to have resistant hypertension [6]. Worth mentioning, resistant hypertension should not be confounded with uncontrolled hypertension, which refers to subjects who fail to reach BP goal with fewer than three drugs or with an inadequate treatment regimen (either by medical inertia or by poor adherence to treatment).

Although current guidelines for the management of resistant hypertension still define resistance to antihypertensive treatment based on OBP measurements, there is increasing awareness of the important limitations that characterize OBP, including the inherent inaccuracy of the technique, the observer's bias and digit preference, a variable interference by the "white-coat effect," and the inability of this approach to collect information on BP during subjects' usual activities and over a long period of time. Despite the availability of more accurate techniques for BP measurement out of the medical office, which might allow overcoming these difficulties, OBP is still considered as the reference standard for the diagnosis of hypertension and for assessment of BP control in treated hypertensive patients [1]. This is likely to occur mainly because most evidence on the cardiovascular risk associated with elevated BP levels as well as on the benefits of BP-lowering treatment has been based on the results of epidemiological studies and clinical trials using OBP [7]. However, analyses of large databases of observational and interventional studies in hypertension implementing ABPM and HBPM in addition to OBP have overwhelmingly shown that a substantial and sometimes larger-than-expected number of subjects initially diagnosed with resistant hypertension or with BP control based on OBP actually correspond to false resistant hypertension (WCRH) and false BP control (MRH) (WCRH) and false BP control (MRH), respectively. Indeed, when considering the threshold values to assess lack of BP control using in-office (OBP ≥140/90 mmHg) and out-of-office techniques (HBP or daytime ABP ≥135/85 mmHg), a treated hypertensive patient may fall into one of four categories: (1) true BP control (normal in-office and out-of-office BP levels); (2) true resistant hypertension (elevated in-office and out-of-office BP levels); (3) false resistant/uncontrolled hypertension (elevated in-office but normal out-of-office BP levels) also known as white-coat resistant/uncontrolled hypertension (WCRH); and (4) false BP control (normal in-office but elevated out-of-office BP levels) also known as masked resistant/uncontrolled hypertension (MRH) (Fig. 6.1).

Although demonstration of elevated office and out-of-office BP levels is an essential step for the diagnosis of true resistant hypertension, several interfering factors other than those related to BP measurement itself (i.e., the "white-coat effect" or cuff-related artifacts) should still be considered before confirming the diagnosis of true resistant hypertension. These include secondary causes of hypertension, inappropriate drug choices or doses, concurrent use of drugs that may interfere with prescribed antihypertensive agents, or failure of the patient to adhere to the prescribed treatment regimen. With regard to this latter issue, several factors may further contribute to discontinuation of antihypertensive treatment increasing the prevalence of false resistant hypertension, such as side effects of multidrug therapy and cost of medications, lack of consistent and continuous primary care, the absence of strong physician motivation, poor understanding of instructions related to treatment, and social and cultural fences. Indeed, recent analyses of several interventional trials have shown that administration of

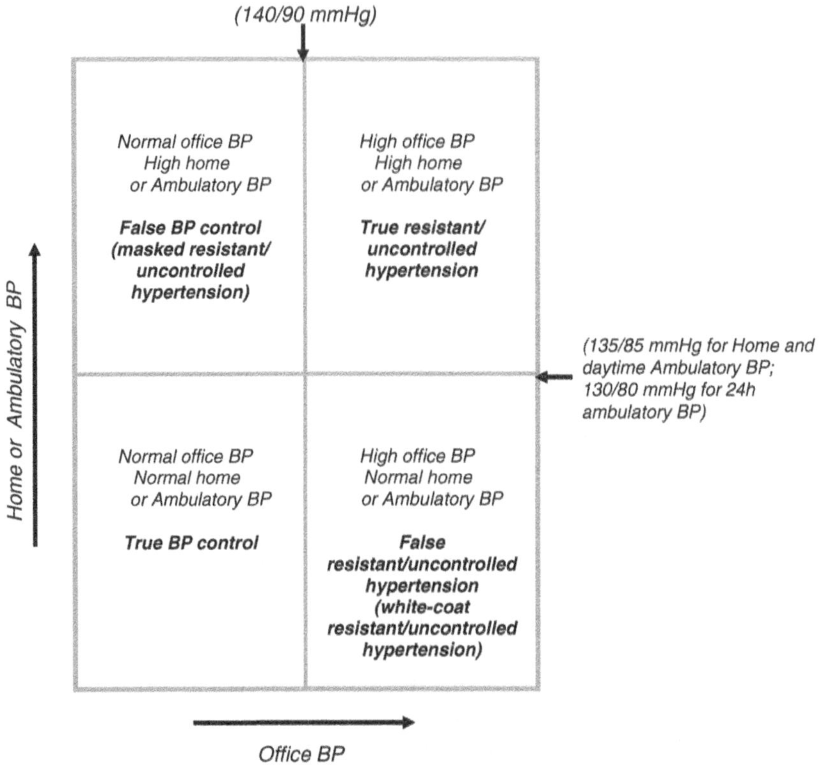

Fig. 6.1 Schematic relationship between office and home or ambulatory BP in treated hypertensive subjects. Classification of patients based on the comparison of office and home or ambulatory blood pressure (*BP*). Modified from Parati et al. [8] with permission

multidrug regimens by clinical staff to subjects who had been previously uncontrolled by antihypertensive treatment resulted in optimal BP control [9], suggesting that in addition to the "white-coat" effect and inaccuracies of OBP measuring techniques, a poor adherence to recommended lifestyle measures and/or drug treatment may be major contributing factors to the apparent resistance to antihypertensive treatment. In some instances, also physicians' inertia may increase the prevalence of false resistant hypertension as indicated by several surveys showing that many physicians not only fail to perform a proper BP measurement in the office but also fail to increase the number of doses of antihypertensive medications as recommended by guidelines when BP levels are out of control.

From a prognostic perspective, a proper assessment of BP control and identification of patients with true resistant hypertension as well as those with MRH (false BP control) are of the highest relevance on the background of the evidence showing these conditions to be associated with a higher prevalence of secondary hypertension and target organ damage [10, 11], as well as with a higher risk of future cardiovascular and renal events, which ultimately translates into greater healthcare costs [6, 12, 13]. Conversely, confirming the achievement of true BP control and excluding the presence of real resistant hypertension by demonstrating adequate out-of-office BP control, through ABPM and/or HBPM, are also important in order to prevent unnecessary modifications to antihypertensive treatment such as inappropriate increase in dosing or number of antihypertensive drugs. This may help reducing the risk of adverse effects associated with multidrug therapy that often interfere with patients' lifestyles affecting compliance. Finally, in recent years, interventional device-based treatment strategies have became available for the management of resistant hypertension (i.e., carotid baroreceptor activation through permanent implantation of a carotid nerve stimulator (Rheos, CVRx, USA) [14] and radiofrequency catheter-based renal denervation [15]). Given the costs and invasive character of these approaches (as well as their potential adverse effects when not properly indicated), an accurate diagnosis of true resistant hypertension based on both office and out-of-office BP measures is currently considered among the eligibility criteria before proceeding with these interventional therapies as recently outlined in a position statement document of the European Society of Hypertension [16].

6.3 Prevalence of True and False Resistant Hypertension ("White-Coat" Resistant Hypertension)

Resistant hypertension is an important medical problem, and its prevalence may substantially differ depending on the population studied and the level of medical screening. In the absence of definitive large prospective epidemiological studies specifically designed to assess the prevalence of this phenomenon, data from large community-based observational studies and clinical trials suggest that about 10 to 30 % of subjects within the overall hypertensive population may be resistant to antihypertensive treatment [3, 17, 18, 19]. The prevalence of resistant hypertension may considerably increase when applying lower BP cutoff limits for defining BP control (i.e., OBP <130/80 mmHg for hypertensive subjects with diabetes mellitus, renal insufficiency, or at high/very high CV risk as previously recommended by guidelines until year 2007). It may also falsely increase due to the presence of the "white-coat" effect, administration of inadequate doses of antihypertensive therapy, improper use of diuretics, and poor adherence to medical treatment after increases in dosing or number of drugs [19, 20]. Of relevance, in a significant proportion of subjects with resistant hypertension, the persistent elevation in OBP has been shown to correspond to WCRH (false resistance hypertension) as indicated by the analysis of observational studies and clinical trials in hypertension [3, 19]. A report from the Spanish Ambulatory Blood Pressure Monitoring Registry provided relevant data on the prevalence and clinical features of resistant hypertension in a large sample of about 68.000 hypertensive patients from Spain who had 24-h ABPM performed and were recruited from primary care and specialty clinics since 2004 [3]. Overall, a total of 8295 subjects, corresponding to 12.2 % of the study population, had resistant hypertension, that is, OBP ≥140/90 mmHg while taking 3 antihypertensive drugs. Interestingly, about 37.5 % of these subjects had relatively normal 24-h ABPM (24-h systolic/diastolic ambulatory BP <130/80 mmHg) so that their elevated OBP could be explained by the "white-coat" effect. This high prevalence of false resistant hypertension exceeds previously reported estimates (18–33 %) of this phenomenon in the general hypertensive population [21]. The remaining 62.5 % of resistant hypertensive subjects in this study had "true resistant hypertension" (i.e., 24-h ABPM ≥130/80 mmHg). More recently, a subsequent report from the Spanish database showed that the prevalence of MRH (false BP control), that is, normal office BP associated with 24-h ambulatory SBP ≥130 and/or DBP ≥80 mmHg, was present in 31 % of treated hypertensive patients apparently controlled based on OBP measures [5]. A previous report on a large sample of Japanese subjects in the frame of the J-HOME Study using cutoff values of 140/90 and 135/85 mmHg for office and home BP, respectively [4], reported a prevalence of WCRH (false resistant hypertension) and true resistant hypertension among patients with resistant hypertension based on office readings of 27.4 and 72.6 %, respectively. Conversely, among patients with controlled OBP, the prevalence of true BP control and MRH (false BP control) was 43.1 and 56.9 %, respectively [4].

In some studies, the clinical characteristics of hypertensive patients with true and false resistant hypertension have been comparatively assessed in an attempt to provide clues to facilitate identification of these two conditions as well as for suggesting strategies and interventions for improving BP management. In a recent report on the National Health and Nutrition Examination Surveys (NHANESs), clinical characteristics associated with apparently treatment-resistant hypertension included ≥4 visits per year, obesity, chronic kidney disease, and Framingham 10-year coronary risk >20 % [22]. In the same line, an analysis of the Spanish registry showed significant differences in the prevalence of CV risk factors between false and true resistant hypertensive patients, the subgroup of subjects with true resistant hypertension being characterized by a significantly higher prevalence of cigarette smoking, diabetes and target organ damage (i.e., left ventricular hypertrophy, microalbuminuria, or impaired renal function), and a history of previous cardiovascular events [3]. However, despite the effort of these studies to identify consistent characteristics and trends in order to distinguish true from false resistant hypertension, the strength of the associations has been very week, being thus unlikely that the differences in risk factor profiles or in selected clinical characteristics might be sufficient to discriminate between these conditions. It must be emphasized that ABPM, ideally accompanied by the use of HBPM for assessment of BP control in the long term, remains the standard method for a correct diagnosis, management, and assessment of BP control of all hypertensive patients not controlled on ≥3 antihypertensive drugs [23].

6.4 In-Office Versus Out-of-Office (ABPM and HBPM) BP Measurement Techniques in Assessing Response to Antihypertensive Treatment

Several interventional studies have shown that the effects of a given BP-lowering strategy (either pharmacological or interventional) on office, and out-of-office BP values, may exhibit substantial quantitative and qualitative differences [24–31]. Evidence on this was provided by a meta-analysis of several studies providing information on drug-induced changes in OBP and 24-h ABPM, comparatively assessing the magnitude of the reduction in office and 24-h ambulatory BP levels induced by antihypertensive treatment [26]. Overall, treatment-induced reductions in 24-h ABPM were found to be smaller than those in systolic (S) and diastolic (D) OBP. While mean reductions in office SBP/DBP were 24.9/14.5 mmHg, those in 24-h ambulatory mean SBP/DBP were 14.6/9.2 mmHg corresponding to about 60 % of the reduction achieved in OBP [26], thus indicating that the effect of antihypertensive treatment is greater on OBP than on ABP. Further confirmation of these findings was provided by a systematic review of literature including data of about 6794 subjects, comparatively assessing the reductions in office versus home and 24-h ambulatory BP levels induced by antihypertensive treatment [27]. Overall, this analysis showed that HBP falls approximately 20 % less than OBP with antihypertensive treatment (mean changes in office and home SBP/DBP were −15.2/−10.3 mmHg and −12.2/−8.0 mmHg, respectively). However, in a study by Ishikawa et al. [27], the reduction in home SBP was greater than that of 24-h SBP (−12.6 mmHg reduction in HBP versus −11.9 mmHg reduction in 24-h SBP; $P < 0.001$). It was also shown that daytime ambulatory SBP falls 15 % less and nighttime systolic BP falls 30 % less than home SBP [27]. Even more striking have been the disagreements observed between in-office and out-of-office BP measuring techniques (either ABPM or HBPM) after interventional procedures (i.e., carotid baroreceptor activation and renal sympathetic denervation) which generally induce marked, direct, and much greater reductions in OBP than those expected with multidrug pharmacological treatment. Indeed, recent systematic reviews of literature have indicated that the reductions in 24-h BP may only correspond to about 30 % of the reductions in OBP induced by interventional strategies, being comparable with the decrease in 24-h BP achieved by conventional treatment [26–31]. Stunningly, in some studies, 24-h ABPM reductions have shown to correspond only to 18 % of the reduction in OBP achieved with interventional strategies, without even reaching statistical significance [32]. The marked disagreements between OBP and out-of-office BP measurement techniques in reflecting the effects of pharmacological and interventional strategies on BP levels have raised serious questions regarding the validity of OBP measures alone not only for assessing BP control during antihypertensive treatment, but also to support the diagnosis of resistant hypertension. It is thought that through their inhibitory effects on sympathetic drive, interventional techniques may induce suppression of the white-coat effect, which in turn might be responsible for the disagreements between OBP and 24-h ABPM. Careful exclusion of patients with WCRH (false resistant hypertension) should thus be a mandatory step for a better evaluation of the actual effects of pharmacological and interventional strategies on BP in future clinical trials [33]. Overall, the above data indicate that OBP readings alone are neither sufficient nor reliable for assessing the response of BP levels to antihypertensive treatment or interventional strategies. A more systematic implementation of ABPM and HBPM is thus needed not only in the setting of interventional trials but also in daily clinical practice, in order to properly assess the actual impact of the tested treatment strategy on BP levels and CV protection.

6.5 Advantages of Out-of-Office BP Measurement Techniques for Assessing BP Control

As shown by observational and interventional studies in treated hypertensives where both in-office and out-of-office BP measurement techniques have been implemented for assessment of BP control, up to one-third of treated hypertensives may be mistakenly classified as having resistant hypertension while they actually show WCRH (false resistant hypertension) [3]. Which is even worse, another 30 % of these subjects may be erroneously classified as having BP controlled, while their out-of-office BP levels actually remain elevated (MRH or false BP control) [4, 5]. Main reasons for these impressive figures include the highly dynamic behavior that characterizes BP levels, which undergo continuous variations over time and the inability of OBP measurements during the medical visit to collect information on BP during subjects' usual activities and over a long period of time. In addition, OBP readings have some limitations related to the inherent inaccuracy of the technique, the observer's bias, and digit preference, as well as a variable interference by the "white-coat effect" due to the alarm reaction generated by the medical visit. A main advantage of out-of-office BP measurements collected either by ABPM or by HBPM is that they allow detection of BP changes in real-life conditions preventing the alarm reaction associated with BP measurement in the medical office responsible for the "white-coat effect,". This, in turn, is considered a major explanation for the frequently observed disagreement between OBP and out-of-office BP measurements [34]. In addition, the use of ABPM allows identification of subjects with alterations in 24-h day-to-night BP changes, that is, non-dippers (subjects with nighttime BP fall <10 %), risers (subjects who have a higher BP during sleep than while awake), or subjects with nocturnal hypertension regardless the degree of day–night BP fall. These abnormal patterns in 24-h ABPM have been reported to occur with a higher frequency among patients with true resistant hypertension [3, 35, 36] and to be associated with an adverse CV prognosis [37–39], which justifies their identification through ABPM as well as targeting antihypertensive treatment toward normalization of ABP profiles. However, despite being considered the gold standard for the diagnosis of hypertension [40, 41] and for assessing BP control in treated hypertensive patients [1, 7], ABPM is costly and is not easily available everywhere. Moreover, it requires trained clinic staff and specialized equipment and may interfere with patients' usual activities and sleep [8]. On the other hand, HBPM shares several of the advantages of ABPM and is less expensive, which supports the current recommendation for its extensive use in clinical practice for the long-term follow-up of BP control in treated hypertensive patients [1, 2, 8, 42]. Nevertheless, at variance from ABPM, self-measurements of BP by patients through HBPM cannot provide the extensive information on daily-life BP behavior available with ambulatory recordings, thus preventing a dynamic assessment of BP within the 24-h period, over daytime, and, in particular, at night. However, when performed on a regular basis, repeated BP measures obtained by patients at home offer the possibility to obtain accurate and frequent information on out-of-office BP not only during a single day, but also over several days, weeks, or months in a usual life setting. This also allows assessing dynamic BP changes (i.e., day-by-day BP variability) over longer periods of time, providing more reliable measures not only on the degree but also on the consistency of BP control over time [8]. Despite its multifold clinical advantages and rapidly growing diffusion, HBPM cannot be considered as an alternative to ABPM, however. Although a major common denominator between HBPM and ABPM is the fact that both of them provide out-of-office BP measurements detecting BP changes in real-life conditions and preventing the alarm reaction associated with OBP [34], they provide complementary (not interchangeable) information on BP in different living conditions and over different periods [8, 40, 43]. The main characteristics of the most important methods for BP measurement in humans are comparatively summarized in Table 6.1.

Table 6.1 modified from Parati et al. [8] by permission. WCH: white-coat hypertension; MH: masked hypertension; OBP: office blood pressure; ABPM: ambulatory BP monitoring; HBPM: home BP monitoring.

Table 6.1 Comparison between features of three main methods for BP measurement

Feature	OBP	ABPM	HBPM
No. of readings	Low	High	Medium
White-coat effect	Yes	No	No
Operator dependency	Yes	No	No
Need of device validation (*Yes if oscillometric device is used)	No*	Yes	Yes
Daytime BP	+	+ + +	+ +
Nighttime BP and dipping (**new HBPM devices may perform nighttime BP measures)	–	+ + +	–/+**
Morning BP	±	+ +	+

(continued)

Table 6.1 (continued)

Feature	OBP	ABPM	HBPM
24-h BP variability	–	+ +	±
Long-term BP variability	–	±	+ +
WCH and MH diagnosis	–	+ +	+ +
Placebo effect	++	–	–
Reproducibility	Low	High (24-h average values)	High (average of several values)
Prognostic value	+	+ + +	+ +
Patient involvement	–	–	+ +
Patient training	–	±	+ +
Physician involvement	+++	++	+
Patients' acceptance	++	±	+ +
Monitoring of treatment effects	Limited information	Extensive information on 24-h BP profile cannot be repeated frequently	Appropriate for long-term monitoring, limited information on 24-h BP profile
Hypertension control improvement	+	++	+++
Cost	Low	High	Low
Availability	High	Low	High

In view of their important advantages, ABPM and HBPM monitoring have been proposed as useful solutions for a better assessment of BP control in treated hypertensive subjects when combined to conventional OBP measurements [34]. This might significantly reduce misclassification of resistant hypertension and better define the need of screening tests for secondary causes of hypertension or implementing more aggressive pharmacological or interventional strategies (i.e., carotid baroreceptor activation or radiofrequency catheter-based renal denervation).

6.6 Identification of True and False Resistant Hypertension (White-Coat Resistant Hypertension) and True and False BP Controls (Masked Uncontrolled/Resistant Hypertension, MRH) in Treated Hypertensives Through ABPM and HBPM

In view of the limitations characterizing OBP measurements, it becomes clear that an adequate assessment of BP control and a proper diagnosis of resistant hypertension cannot be based on isolated OBP readings only. Considering the high prevalence of WCRH (false resistant hypertension) among subjects with resistant hypertension, a practical approach to facilitate the diagnostic evaluation of resistant hypertension consists in classifying patients into two wide categories: true resistance hypertension and false resistance hypertension. Thus, a first step in the evaluation of the patient with a diagnosis of resistant hypertension (made on the basis of OBP measurements) consists in confirming the presence of true resistance to treatment by the combined use of office and out-of-office BP measurement techniques, and thus in excluding WCRH. As mentioned above, ABPM and HBPM provide out-of-office BP measurements detecting BP changes in real-life conditions preventing the alarm reaction associated with OBP [34] which is considered a major contributor to the frequently observed disagreement between OBP and out-of-office BP measurements (Fig. 6.1).

In untreated populations, the prognostic relevance of white-coat hypertension (WCH, elevated OBP, and normal ABP or HBP) is still debated, although it seems to modestly increase CV risk [44]. On the contrary, identification of masked hypertension (normal OBP and elevated ABP or HBP levels) [45, 46] is important on the background of the evidence showing MH to be associated with an elevated CV risk, close to that of patients with sustained hypertension (in whom, both OBP and out-of-office BPs are elevated) [47–49]. In treated hypertensive subjects, identifying true and MRH (false BP control) is of outmost importance on the background of the evidence showing an elevated risk of target organ damage (i.e., left ventricular hypertrophy and microalbuminuria) [10, 11] as well as an increased incidence of fatal and non-fatal cardiovascular events in these subjects when compared to those with true BP control [50–52].

Although MH was first studied with ABPM [45], recent studies have indicated that HBPM is as reliable as ABPM in identifying this phenomenon as well as the associated target organ damage associated with MH [53] although ABPM and HBPM may not necessarily identify the same patients with MH, given that they obtain information on different components of daily life BP. Indeed, during the initial diagnostic approach to hypertension, HBPM may be useful in identifying "truly" hypertensive patients, likely to benefit from implementation of antihypertensive therapy [54]. Evidence on the diagnostic value of HBPM for discriminating between true and false resistant hypertensions has also been provided in a recent study conducted in a group of subjects on stable treatment with $\geq$3 antihypertensive drugs using ABPM as reference method [55]. Office resistant hypertension was defined as elevated OBP ($\geq$140/90 mmHg) and true resistant hypertension as concomitant elevation in office and out-of-office BP (SBP and/or DBP $\geq$135/85 mmHg for HBP or awake ABP). There was agreement between ABP and HBP in confirming clinic resistant hypertension in 82 % of the cases (59 % with and 23 % without true resistant hypertension; kappa 0.59). Regarding the diagnosis of true resistant hypertension, there was agreement between ABP and HBP in 74 % of the cases (49 % with and 25 % without true resistant hypertension; kappa 0.46). The sensitivity, specificity, and positive and negative predictive values for HBP in confirming clinic resistant hypertension were 93, 63, 81, and 83 %, respectively. The respective values for HBP in detecting true resistant

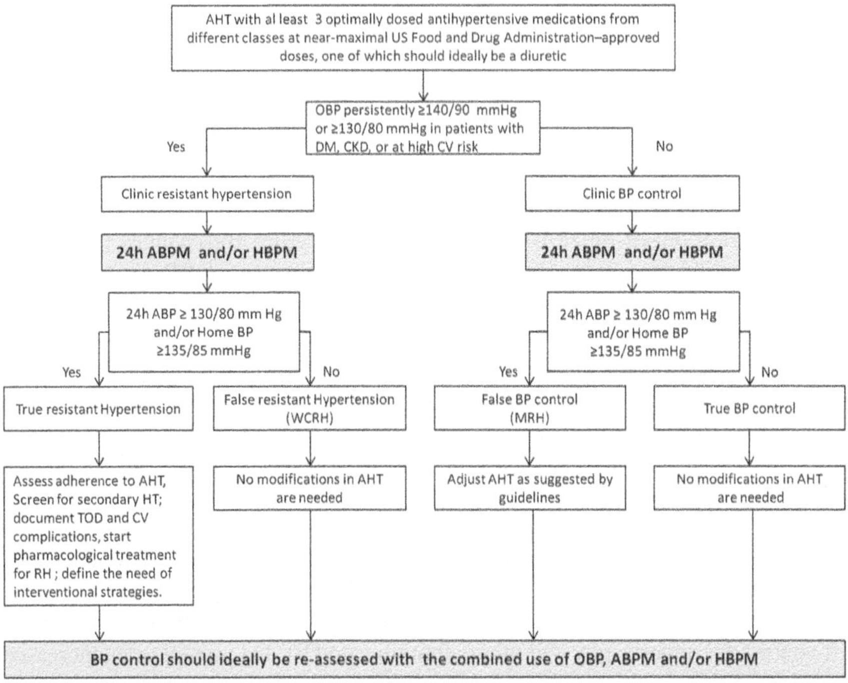

Fig. 6.2 Initial diagnostic approach to the patient with clinic resistant hypertension. *AHT* antihypertensive treatment, *HT* hypertension, *OBP* office blood pressure, *DM* diabetes mellitus, *CKD* chronic kidney disease, *CV* cardiovascular, *BP* blood pressure, *ABPM* ambulatory blood pressure monitoring, *HBPM* home blood pressure monitoring, *WCRH* "white-coat" resistant hypertension, *MRH* "masked" resistant hypertension, *RH* resistant hypertension

hypertension were 90 %, 55 %, 71, and 82 %, indicating that HBP may be a reliable alternative to ABPM in the evaluation of resistant hypertension [55].

Based on the above data, it may be concluded that a proper assessment of BP control and classification of treated hypertensive patients with the combined use of office, ambulatory, and ideally home BP measurements are essential for defining the need for performing additional diagnostic procedures (i.e., screening tests for secondary causes of resistant hypertension) and/or implementing more aggressive pharmacological or interventional strategies. (Fig. 6.2).

6.7 Conclusions

Because false resistant hypertension may be present in a substantial and higher-than-expected number of treated hypertensive patients, confirmation of true resistance to antihypertensive treatment in daily life is a key step during the diagnostic approach to patients who present with persistently elevated clinic BP levels despite properly administered antihypertensive regimen. Although some studies have identified significant differences in the prevalence of some clinical characteristics and cardiovascular risk factors between subjects with false and true resistant hypertensions, the strength of the associations has been week, being thus unlikely that these clinical characteristics are sufficient to discriminate between these diagnoses. It must be emphasized that at present, ABPM remains the standard method for management and assessment of BP control and for a correct diagnosis of resistant hypertension in all hypertensive patients not controlled in the clinic on ≥3 antihypertensive drugs [23]. In addition, ABPM provides information about the circadian patterns of BP, in particular on the degree of day-to-night BP reduction which is frequently blunted or even inverted in subjects with resistant hypertension. Although ABPM is considered the reference method to characterize different subtypes of resistant hypertension, a recent study showed that also HBPM may provide reliable information to discriminate between false and true resistant hypertensions and between true and false BP control, thus reducing misclassification of treated hypertensive subjects [55]. At variance from ABPM which only provides information on BP levels within the 24-h period, a proper implementation of HBPM offers the possibility to perform accurate and frequent out-of-office BP measurements not only during a single day, but also over several days, weeks, or months in a usual life setting, thus allowing a better assessment of the degree and consistency of BP response to antihypertensive treatment in the long term. Indeed, the use of HBPM has been strongly supported by current guidelines for assessment of BP control in treated patients in whom a proper assessment of the degree and consistency of BP reduction over time are necessary [1, 2], on the background of the evidence that ABPM and HBPM provide complementary and not redundant information on BP levels. Once the diagnosis of true resistant hypertension has been confirmed, further steps include assessment of adherence to antihypertensive treatment, screening for identifiable causes of hypertension (i.e., hyperaldosteronism, obstructive sleep apnea, chronic kidney disease, renal artery stenosis, and pheochromocytoma), documentation of target organ damage and CV complications, and defining the need to intensify pharmacological treatment versus performing interventional strategies. Whenever possible, subjects with confirmed resistant hypertension should ideally be referred to a hypertension specialist [6]. Conversely, confirmation of false resistant hypertension may avoid unnecessary and costly additional diagnostic tests, also preventing from improperly increasing doses or number of medications and thus reducing the associated adverse effects of multidrug therapy. Finally, as shown by several meta-analyses of observational and interventional studies, OBP alone is unreliable either to support the diagnosis of resistant hypertension or for assessing BP control, following pharmacological or interventional strategies. Despite all the above evidence, in clinical practice, the efficacy of BP-lowering strategies is still often assessed just based on office BP without considering ambulatory and home BP measurements. For a better assessment of the actual benefits of these strategies not only in terms of BP control but also in relation to their impact on cardiovascular prognosis, forthcoming studies implementing the combined use of office, ambulatory, and home BP measures are necessary.

References

1. Mancia G, De Backer G, Dominiczak A, Cifkova R, Fagard R, Germano G, Grassi G, Heagerty AM, Kjeldsen SE, Laurent S et al (2007) Guidelines for the management of arterial hypertension: the task force for the management of arterial hypertension of the European Society of Hypertension (ESH) and of the European Society of Cardiology (ESC). J Hypertens 25(6):1105–1187
2. Chobanian AV, Bakris GL, Black HR, Cushman WC, Green LA, Izzo JL Jr, Jones DW, Materson BJ, Oparil S, Wright JT Jr et al (2003) Seventh report of the joint national committee on prevention, detection, evaluation, and treatment of high blood pressure. Hypertension 42(6):1206–1252
3. de la Sierra A, Segura J, Banegas JR, Gorostidi M, de la Cruz JJ, Armario P, Oliveras A, Ruilope LM (2011) Clinical features of 8295 patients with resistant hypertension classified on the basis of ambulatory blood pressure monitoring. Hypertension 57(5):898–902
4. Oikawa T, Obara T, Ohkubo T, Kikuya M, Asayama K, Metoki H, Komai R, Murai K, Hashimoto J, Totsune K et al (2006) Characteristics of resistant hypertension determined by self-measured blood pressure at home and office blood pressure measurements: the J-HOME study. J Hypertens 24(9):1737–1743
5. de la Sierra A, Banegas JR, Oliveras A, Gorostidi M, Segura J, de la Cruz JJ, Armario P, Ruilope LM (2012) Clinical differences between resistant hypertensives and patients treated and controlled with three or less drugs. J Hypertens 30(6):1211–1216
6. Calhoun DA, Jones D, Textor S, Goff DC, Murphy TP, Toto RD, White A, Cushman WC, White W, Sica D et al (2008) Resistant hypertension: diagnosis, evaluation, and treatment. A scientific statement from the American Heart Association Professional Education Committee of the council for high blood pressure research. Hypertension 51(6):1403–1419
7. O'Brien E, Asmar R, Beilin L, Imai Y, Mallion JM, Mancia G, Mengden T, Myers M, Padfield P, Palatini P et al (2003) European Society of Hypertension recommendations for conventional, ambulatory and home blood pressure measurement. J Hypertens 21(5):821–848
8. Parati G, Stergiou GS, Asmar R, Bilo G, de Leeuw P, Imai Y, Kario K, Lurbe E, Manolis A, Mengden T et al (2008) European society of hypertension guidelines for blood pressure monitoring at home: a summary report of the second international consensus conference on home blood pressure monitoring. J Hypertens 26(8):1505–1526
9. Bunker J, Callister W, Chang CL, Sever PS (2011) How common is true resistant hypertension? J Hum Hypertens 25(2):137–140
10. Muxfeldt ES, Bloch KV, Nogueira Ada R, Salles GF (2005) True resistant hypertension: is it possible to be recognized in the office? American j hypertens 18(12 Pt 1):1534–1540
11. Oliveras A, Armario P, Hernandez-Del Rey R, Arroyo JA, Poch E, Larrousse M, Roca-Cusachs A, de la Sierra A (2010) Urinary albumin excretion is associated with true resistant hypertension. J Hum Hypertens 24(1):27–33
12. Cuspidi C, Macca G, Sampieri L, Michev I, Salerno M, Fusi V, Severgnini B, Meani S, Magrini F, Zanchetti A (2001) High prevalence of cardiac and extracardiac target organ damage in refractory hypertension. J Hypertens 19(11):2063–2070
13. Moser M, Setaro JF (2006) Clinical practice. Resistant or difficult-to-control hypertension. The New England j med 355(4):385–392
14. Papademetriou V, Doumas M, Faselis C, Tsioufis C, Douma S, Gkaliagkousi E, Zamboulis C (2011) Carotid baroreceptor stimulation for the treatment of resistant hypertension. Int j hypertens 2011:964394
15. Doumas M, Faselis C, Papademetriou V (2011) Renal sympathetic denervation in hypertension. Curr Opin Nephrol Hypertens 20(6):647–653
16. Schmieder RE, Redon J, Grassi G, Kjeldsen SE, Mancia G, Narkiewicz K, Parati G, Ruilope L, van de Borne P, Tsioufis C (2012) ESH position paper: renal denervation—an interventional therapy of resistant hypertension. J Hypertens 30(5):837–841

17. Cushman WC, Ford CE, Cutler JA, Margolis KL, Davis BR, Grimm RH, Black HR, Hamilton BP, Holland J, Nwachuku C et al (2002) Success and predictors of blood pressure control in diverse North American settings: the antihypertensive and lipid-lowering treatment to prevent heart attack trial (ALLHAT). J Clin Hypertens (Greenwich) 4(6):393–404
18. Hajjar I, Kotchen TA (2003) Trends in prevalence, awareness, treatment, and control of hypertension in the United States, 1988–2000. JAMA, J Am Med Assoc 290(2):199–206
19. Persell SD (2011) Prevalence of resistant hypertension in the United States, 2003–2008. Hypertension 57(6):1076–1080
20. Ahmed MI, Calhoun DA (2011) Resistant hypertension: bad and getting worse. Hypertension 57(6):1045–1046
21. Elliott WJ (2011) High prevalence of white-coat hypertension in Spanish resistant hypertensive patients. Hypertension 57(5):889–890
22. Egan BM, Zhao Y, Axon RN, Brzezinski WA, Ferdinand KC (2011) Uncontrolled and apparent treatment resistant hypertension in the United States, 1988–2008. Circulation 124(9):1046–1058
23. O'Brien E (2008) Ambulatory blood pressure measurement: the case for implementation in primary care. Hypertension 51(6):1435–1441
24. Mancia G, Parati G, Bilo G, Maronati A, Omboni S, Baurecht H, Hennig M, Zanchetti A (2007) Assessment of long-term antihypertensive treatment by clinic and ambulatory blood pressure: data from the European lacidipine study on atherosclerosis. J Hypertens 25(5):1087–1094
25. Mancia G, Omboni S, Parati G, Clement DL, Haley WE, Rahman SN, Hoogma RP (2001) Twenty-four hour ambulatory blood pressure in the hypertension optimal treatment (HOT) study. J Hypertens 19(10):1755–1763
26. Mancia G, Parati G (2004) Office compared with ambulatory blood pressure in assessing response to antihypertensive treatment: a meta-analysis. J Hypertens 22(3):435–445
27. Ishikawa J, Carroll DJ, Kuruvilla S, Schwartz JE, Pickering TG (2008) Changes in home versus clinic blood pressure with antihypertensive treatments: a meta-analysis. Hypertension 52(5):856–864
28. Scheffers IJ, Kroon AA, Schmidli J, Jordan J, Tordoir JJ, Mohaupt MG, Luft FC, Haller H, Menne J, Engeli S et al (2010) Novel baroreflex activation therapy in resistant hypertension: results of a European multi-center feasibility study. J Am Coll Cardiol 56(15):1254–1258
29. Bakris GL, Lindholm LH, Black HR, Krum H, Linas S, Linseman JV, Arterburn S, Sager P, Weber M (2010) Divergent results using clinic and ambulatory blood pressures: report of a darusentan-resistant hypertension trial. Hypertension 56(5):824–830
30. Krum H, Schlaich M, Whitbourn R, Sobotka PA, Sadowski J, Bartus K, Kapelak B, Walton A, Sievert H, Thambar S et al (2009) Catheter-based renal sympathetic denervation for resistant hypertension: a multicentre safety and proof-of-principle cohort study. Lancet 373(9671):1275–1281
31. Esler MD, Krum H, Sobotka PA, Schlaich MP, Schmieder RE, Bohm M (2010) Renal sympathetic denervation in patients with treatment-resistant hypertension (The Symplicity HTN-2 Trial): a randomised controlled trial. Lancet 376(9756):1903–1909
32. Witkowski A, Prejbisz A, Florczak E, Kadziela J, Sliwinski P, Bielen P, Michalowska I, Kabat M, Warchol E, Januszewicz M et al (2011) Effects of renal sympathetic denervation on blood pressure, sleep apnea course, and glycemic control in patients with resistant hypertension and sleep apnea. Hypertension 58(4):559–565
33. Doumas M, Anyfanti P, Bakris G (2012) Should ambulatory blood pressure monitoring be mandatory for future studies in resistant hypertension: a perspective. J Hypertens 30(5):874–876
34. Asayama K, Ohkubo T, Kikuya M, Metoki H, Obara T, Hoshi H, Hashimoto J, Totsune K, Satoh H, Imai Y (2005) Use of 2003 European society of hypertension-European society of cardiology guidelines for predicting stroke using self-measured blood pressure at home: the Ohasama study. Eur Heart J 26(19):2026–2031

35. Muxfeldt ES, Cardoso CR, Salles GF (2009) Prognostic value of nocturnal blood pressure reduction in resistant hypertension. Arch Intern Med 169(9):874–880
36. Muxfeldt ES, Bloch KV, Nogueira AR, Salles GF (2003) Twenty-four hour ambulatory blood pressure monitoring pattern of resistant hypertension. Blood Press Monit 8(5):181–185
37. de la Sierra A, Redon J, Banegas JR, Segura J, Parati G, Gorostidi M, de la Cruz JJ, Sobrino J, Llisterri JL, Alonso J et al (2009) Prevalence and factors associated with circadian blood pressure patterns in hypertensive patients. Hypertension 53(3):466–472
38. Staessen JA, Thijs L, Fagard R, O'Brien ET, Clement D, de Leeuw PW, Mancia G, Nachev C, Palatini P, Parati G et al (1999) Predicting cardiovascular risk using conventional vs ambulatory blood pressure in older patients with systolic hypertension. Systolic hypertension in Europe trial investigators. JAMA, J Am Med Assoc 282(6):539–546
39. Verdecchia P (2000) Prognostic value of ambulatory blood pressure: current evidence and clinical implications. Hypertension 35(3):844–851
40. Pickering TG, Miller NH, Ogedegbe G, Krakoff LR, Artinian NT, Goff D (2008) Call to action on use and reimbursement for home blood pressure monitoring: a joint scientific statement from the American Heart Association, American society of hypertension, and preventive cardiovascular nurses association. Hypertension 52(1):10–29
41. Ritchie LD, Campbell NC, Murchie P (2011) New NICE guidelines for hypertension. BMJ 343:d5644
42. Parati G, Stergiou GS, Asmar R, Bilo G, de Leeuw P, Imai Y, Kario K, Lurbe E, Manolis A, Mengden T et al (2010) European Society of Hypertension practice guidelines for home blood pressure monitoring. J Hum Hypertens 24(12):779–785
43. Parati G, Bilo G (2009) Home blood pressure measurements will or will not replace 24-hour ambulatory blood pressure measurement. Hypertension
44. Ohkubo T, Kikuya M, Metoki H, Asayama K, Obara T, Hashimoto J, Totsune K, Hoshi H, Satoh H, Imai Y (2005) Prognosis of "masked" hypertension and "white-coat" hypertension detected by 24-h ambulatory blood pressure monitoring 10-year follow-up from the Ohasama study. J Am Coll Cardiol 46(3):508–515
45. Pickering TG, Davidson K, Gerin W, Schwartz JE (2002) Masked hypertension. Hypertension 40(6):795–796
46. Parati G, Ulian L, Santucciu C, Omboni S, Mancia G (1998) Difference between clinic and daytime blood pressure is not a measure of the white coat effect. Hypertension 31(5):1185–1189
47. Mancia G, Facchetti R, Bombelli M, Grassi G, Sega R (2006) Long-term risk of mortality associated with selective and combined elevation in office, home, and ambulatory blood pressure. Hypertension 47(5):846–853
48. Bobrie G, Chatellier G, Genes N, Clerson P, Vaur L, Vaisse B, Menard J, Mallion JM (2004) Cardiovascular prognosis of "masked hypertension" detected by blood pressure self-measurement in elderly treated hypertensive patients. JAMA, J Am Med Assoc 291(11):1342–1349
49. Fagard RH, Celis H, Thijs L, Staessen JA, Clement DL, De Buyzere ML, De Bacquer DA (2008) Daytime and nighttime blood pressure as predictors of death and cause-specific cardiovascular events in hypertension. Hypertension 51(1):55–61
50. Pierdomenico SD, Lapenna D, Bucci A, Di Tommaso R, Di Mascio R, Manente BM, Caldarella MP, Neri M, Cuccurullo F, Mezzetti A (2005) Cardiovascular outcome in treated hypertensive patients with responder, masked, false resistant, and true resistant hypertension. Am J Hypertens 18(11):1422–1428
51. Redon J, Campos C, Narciso ML, Rodicio JL, Pascual JM, Ruilope LM (1998) Prognostic value of ambulatory blood pressure monitoring in refractory hypertension: a prospective study. Hypertension 31(2):712–718
52. Salles GF, Cardoso CR, Muxfeldt ES (2008) Prognostic influence of office and ambulatory blood pressures in resistant hypertension. Arch Intern Med 168(21):2340–2346

53. Stergiou GS, Salgami EV, Tzamouranis DG, Roussias LG (2005) Masked hypertension assessed by ambulatory blood pressure versus home blood pressure monitoring: is it the same phenomenon? Am J Hypertens 18(6):772–778
54. Staessen JA, Den Hond E, Celis H, Fagard R, Keary L, Vandenhoven G, O'Brien ET (2004) Antihypertensive treatment based on blood pressure measurement at home or in the physician's office: a randomized controlled trial. JAMA, J Am Med Assoc 291(8):955–964
55. Nasothimiou EG, Tzamouranis D, Roussias LG, Stergiou GS (2011) Home versus ambulatory blood pressure monitoring in the diagnosis of clinic resistant and true resistant hypertension. J Human Hypertens

7 Causes of Resistant Hypertension

Roland E. Schmieder

7.1 Pseudohypertension

Pseudohypertension is defined as factitious lack of blood pressure (BP) control caused by inaccurate measurement of BP to flawed measurements or due to the 'white-coat' effect. Identification of pseudohypertension avoids overtreatment, potential side effects by additional (unnecessary) medication, and excessive and expensive evaluation of drug therapy [1, 2].

7.1.1 'White-Coat' Effect/'White-Coat' Hypertension

'White-coat' effect is the difference between office BP and ambulatory or home BP measurements and can be calculated as the mean office BP minus mean daytime ambulatory BP [3]. This phenomenon is common, with a prevalence of 20–30 % among patients with hypertension. Elderly individuals tend to exhibit more 'white-coat' effects than younger individuals [4, 5]. In clinical practice, patients who are experiencing the 'white-coat' effect may be identified through the use of out-of-office BP monitoring techniques. Currently, there are two modalities that provide out-of-office BP measurements that are used in clinical practice: 24-h ambulatory BP monitoring (ABPM) and self or home BP monitoring.

R. E. Schmieder (✉)
Nephrology and Hypertension, University Hospital Erlangen, Ulmenweg 18, 91054 Erlangen, Germany
e-mail: roland.schmieder@uk-erlangen.de

G. Mancia (ed.), *Resistant Hypertension*, DOI: 10.1007/978-88-470-5415-8_7,

7.1.2 Pseudohypertension

Falsely increased BP may result from markedly sclerotic arteries which do not collapse during inflation of the BP cuff. In the elderly, the brachial arteries may become very thickened and stiff due to arterial medial sclerosis and calcification. Although the Osler's maneuver has been recommended as a means of screening for pseudohypertension [6], investigators have reported it to have questionable accuracy and usefulness [7]. Correct identification of pseudohypertension is necessary to avoid overtreating hypertensive patients and should be suspected in elderly or diabetic patients with refractory hypertension and in those without organ damage and/or symptoms of overmedication [8]. Confirmation of pseudohypertension requires direct intra-arterial measurement of BP, and differences up to 50 mmHg have been reported in individual elderly hypertensive patients [6, 9].
Question for the daily work: Has white-coat effect been ruled out?
Diagnostic instrument: Evaluate home and/or ambulatory BP measurements

7.2 Renal Hypertension

7.2.1 Renal Artery Stenosis

Hemodynamically relevant renal artery stenosis (RAS) is found in a substantial portion of patients with treatment-resistant hypertension [10]. The prevalence of RAS ranges from 4 to 50 % in autopsy studies and is approximately 10 % according to clinical studies [1, 10, 11]. Its prevalence increases with age due to the progressive nature of atherosclerosis. Although several methods are used for the detection of RAS with rather good sensitivity and specificity, the diagnosis of secondary hypertension often represents an unfulfilled challenge for GPs and referral in specialized centers is required to definitively rule out RAS.

Stenotic lesions are largely secondary to atherosclerosis (90 %) [10]. These patients have to be evaluated with renal artery Doppler ultrasonography, magnetic resonance angiography, or computed tomography scan (be aware of radiation exposure) of the renal arteries [12, 13]. The renal venous–renin ratio is the only diagnostic procedure able to determine renin production of each kidney separately and can be of considerable assistance in treatment decision making, but its use is decreasing due to low sensitivity and its invasive procedure. Nevertheless, it was found to predict improvement of hypertension after nephrectomy in patients suspected of having unilateral renal renin hypersecretion associated with ipsilateral marked or complete loss of kidney function [14, 15].

Fibromuscular dysplasia is a much less frequent cause of RAS (approximately 10 %), is more frequently found in younger and female patients [10, 16], and can be successfully treated by percutaneous dilatation [17].

Screening test for renal artery disease: duplex ultrasonography, magnetic resonance angiography

7.2.2 Renal Parenchymal Disease

Chronic renal failure frequently not only causes resistant hypertension but is also a frequent complication of arterial hypertension in the sense of hypertensive end-organ damage. The bidirectional pathomechanism between renal failure and hypertension may explain why fewer than 15 % of patients with chronic renal disease achieve the target value of <130/80 mm Hg despite taking a combination of three or more medications [1]. All so far published guidelines recommend lower blood pressure goals in patients with chronic kidney disease, especially when overt proteinuria albuminuria is present [18].

Albuminuria and glomerular filtration rate are baseline diagnostic procedures indicating not only renal but also cardiovascular risk and need be assessed in all patients with resistant hypertension. Increases in serum creatinine occur at a late stage of kidney disease. Glomerular filtration rate should be estimated by the use of the Modification of Diet in Renal Disease (MDRD) Study, the CKD-EPI formula, or Cockcroft–Gault equation [19].

Screening test for renal parenchymal disease: Urine analysis (stick test, microscopic analysis of the urine, e.g., erythrocytes?), quantification of albuminuria and proteinuria (urinary albumin creatinine ratio in the spot urine), estimated glomerular filtration rate (eGFR)

Findings: red blood cells, (acanthocytes), albuminuria >30 mg/g *creatinine (microalbuminuria), proteinuria* >1 g/day, *eGFR* < 60 ml/min/1.73 m^2

7.3 Endocrine Causes of Secondary Hypertension

7.3.1 Primary Hyperaldosteronism

Primary hyperaldosteronism is the most common cause of secondary hypertension and is a frequent contributor to treatment resistance [20, 21]. Around 10 % (to 20 %) of patients with resistant arterial hypertension have primary hyperaldosteronism [21]. Although the diagnosis of adrenal adenomas prevailed during older times, recent reports reveal that hyperplasia is more frequent than adrenal adenomas [21, 22]. The adenoma is usually unilateral and is comprised of glomerulosa cells in the adrenal cortex. Primary hyperaldosteronism is rarely caused by adrenal carcinoma.

Diagnosis is suspected in patients with hypertension with persistent hypokalemia or normokalemia in the lower normal range. The screening tool in these patients is elevated plasma aldosterone levels related to low plasma renin activity (PRA), without interaction of drugs that profoundly affect the hormone levels (in particular aldosterone antagonists, direct renin inhibitors). The prevalence of hyperaldosteronism is much greater than previously thought, partially because hypokalemia and adrenal tumors are no longer necessary criteria for the diagnosis. Of course, the telltale symptom is hypokalemia, although up to 50 % of patients with confirmed primary hyperaldosteronism display normal potassium [23]. The prevalence is positively correlated with the severity of BP [24]: Among untreated patients, the prevalence of hyperaldosteronism increases with increasing severity of hypertension, from 2 % in patients with stage 1 hypertension to 8 % in those with stage 2 hypertension and 13 % in those with stage 3 hypertension [25]. The prevalence is even higher in patients with resistant hypertension, approaching 17–22 % in studies [23, 26].

In a prospective study, 20 % of patients with resistant hypertension were diagnosed with primary hyperaldosteronism based on a suppressed plasma renin activity (<1.0 ng/mL/h) and a high 24-hour urinary aldosterone excretion (>12 µg/24 h) during high dietary sodium intake (>200 mEq/24 h) [23]. Because of its high prevalence in this patient group, all patients with resistant hypertension, even those with normal potassium levels, should be evaluated for primary hyperaldosteronism [21, 26, 27].

Aldosterone–renin ratio is considered the most reliable test for screening primary hyperaldosteronism, but false-positive and false-negative results may occur depending on posture, time of the day, salt intake, plasma potassium, and concurrent medications [28]. Interfering medications should be ideally stopped before screening for primary hyperaldosteronism. However, the risk of stopping medications in patients with resistant hypertension needs to be carefully assessed in order to avoid loss of hypertension control. The impact of concomitant medication is small by the use of α-blockers, such as doxazosin, and ACE inhibitors, such as fosinopril, on the aldosterone–renin ratio [29]. Amlodipine, a calcium channel blocker, gave only a small percentage of false-negative diagnoses, suggesting that it could be used if strictly necessary to control blood pressure. ß-Blockers also do not substantially interfere with the diagnosis of primary hyperaldosteronism, but they could be responsible for an increased rate of false-positive ratio and therefore of an increased necessity for the confirmatory test of hyperaldosteronism [28, 29]. Of course, aldosterone antagonists (spironolactone, eplerenone) and direct renin inhibitor aliskiren (false measurements of serum renin concentrations) need to be stopped at all events.

If aldosterone–renin ratio is positive, primary hyperaldosteronism has to be confirmed by fludrocortisone suppression test or oral sodium loading/saline infusion testing [20]. After confirmation, lateralization of the source of the excessive aldosterone secretion demonstrated by adrenal vein sampling is critical to guide the management of primary hyperaldosteronism [20, 27, 28], but bilateral venous blood sampling is a challenging procedure and success rate is approximately 75 % at best [30].

The other forms of endocrine hypertension, presented in Fig. (7.1), are less frequently encountered in hypertensive patients and, therefore, represent more rare causes of resistant hypertension. In addition, the clinical presentation of these endocrine forms of secondary hypertension is usually so characteristic that is really difficult to miss them.

Screening test for aldosteronism: *ARR* (*aldosterone–renin ratio*)
Signs: Elevated ARR (*depending on laboratory methods*)

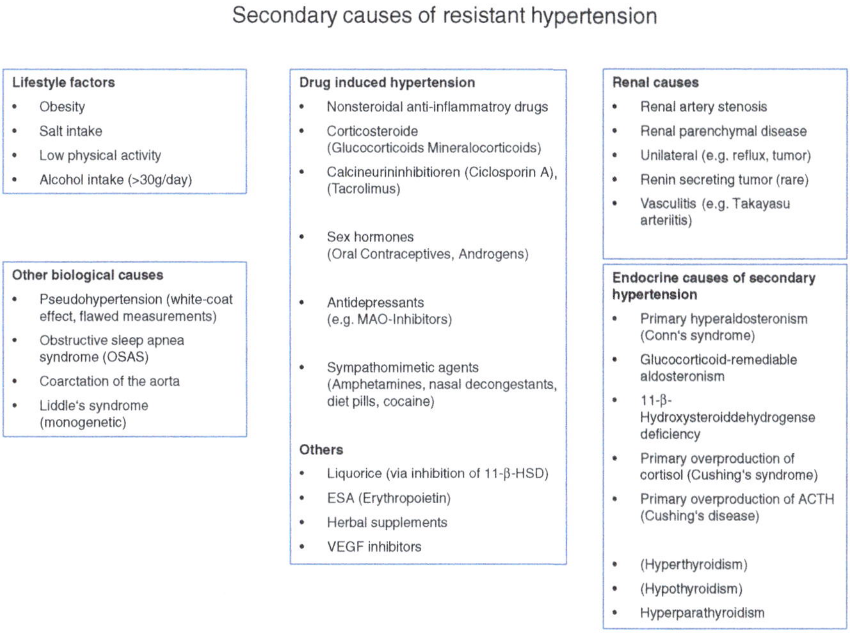

Fig. 7.1 Secondary causes of hypertension

Screening test for Cushing's syndrome: Urinary free cortisol (UFC), dexamethasone suppression test

Signs: Increased 24-h *UFC level*: 3–4 *times upper limit of the normal range* (40–50 μg/24 h), *lack of cortisol suppression* (*morning plasma cortisol levels* >1.8 μg/dl)

7.3.2 Pheochromocytoma

Although the prevalence of pheochromocytoma in the general hypertensive population is very low (0.1–0.6 %) [31, 32], the diagnosis and treatment are extremely important due to hypertensive crisis if the tumor is stimulated and the possibility that the tumor could be malignant. The clinical presentation of pheochromocytoma is widely variable, but the triad of headache, palpitations, and sweating are the most common findings [32]. Of note, only 50 % have episodes of hypertensive crisis, and the other half have committedly elevated BP.

All patients with resistant hypertension and symptoms typical of pheochromocytoma should be screened. Plasma-free metanephrines are the best screening test for pheochromocytoma, with high sensitivity (99 %) and specificity (89 %) [32]. Surgical removal of the tumor is the appropriate treatment.

Screening test for pheochromocytoma: Urine tests for catecholamine hypersecretion

Signs: For urinary catecholamines, total metanephrines: >1.3 g/24 h (*depending on laboratory method*)

7.3.3 Hyperthyroidism/Hypothyroidism

In a study of nearly 700 patients (ages 15–70 years) referred for hypertension management, nearly 4 % were found to have unrecognized hyperthyroidism, whereas 3.6 % had serum levels indicative of hypothyroidism [33, 34]. Although the prevalence of hypertension increases with age, none of the studies reported an age-related increase in the prevalence of hypertension with hyperthyroidism [33, 34].

Hypertension incidence increased with age in both euthyroid and hypothyroid women with thyroiditis, but hypothyroid patients had significantly greater diastolic blood pressure in the fifth and sixth decades of life than did euthyroid controls [34].

In general, it is not recommended to screen for hyper- or hypothyroidism in resistant hypertension, unless clinical symptoms indicate severe alteration in the thyroid gland.

Screening test for hyperthyroidism and hypothyroidism: TSH test (if indicated).

Signs: Abnormal serum TSH level is a sensitive indicator of change in thyroid function.

7.4 Poor Adherence to Therapeutic Plan

7.4.1 Obesity

Increased body weight is often associated with increased BP, and blood pressure control is more difficult to achieve in obese than in lean hypertensive patients. Due to the positive correlation between body mass index and blood pressure, it is well accepted that weight loss results in blood pressure reduction [18, 35]. Patients who are overweight or obese should be counseled to lose weight, ideally attaining a body mass index (BMI) <25 kg/m^2. By and large 1 kg body weight reduction is associated with an average reduction in BP of 2/1 mm Hg [35]. The relation appeared to be linear.

Nevertheless, it is important to stress that the need for weight loss should not be used as a reason to delay pharmacologic therapy in patients with hypertension. Rather, pharmacologic therapy should be used to control BP until lifestyle changes take effect, at which time antihypertensive medication may be reduced. Weight loss can be a big and often frustrating challenge for many patients. Powerful cultural forces, social norms, and commercial interests encourage a sedentary lifestyle, suboptimal diet, and overconsumption of calories. Even motivated patients may find it difficult to sustain behavioral changes in diet and exercise [36].

Question for the daily work: Is the patient obese and/or has weight gained recently?

Therapeutic instrument: Discuss diet and lifestyle changes according to the patient's possibilities.

7.4.2 Salt Intake

The average adult male in the western hemisphere consumes 10–14 g salt per day. This is significantly higher than the recommended daily salt intake of <5–6 g/day (2–2,4 sodium/day) [18, 37]. Excessive sodium intake contributes to treatment-resistant hypertension and increases stroke, left ventricular hypertrophy, and proteinuria independent of blood pressure [37]. Conversely, a decrease in salt intake of 12 g/day was associated with fall in blood pressure by approximately 20/10 mm Hg (Fig. 7.2) [38].

The response to dietary salt reduction is heterogeneous, but black and older-aged patients tend to be more sensitive to the effects of sodium on BP [35, 37]. Individuals with hypertension, diabetes, or chronic kidney disease also display greater sodium sensitivity. On average, BP increases with increased sodium consumption, but there is no practical diagnostic test to distinguish a salt-sensitive individual from one who is less sensitive to the effects of sodium.

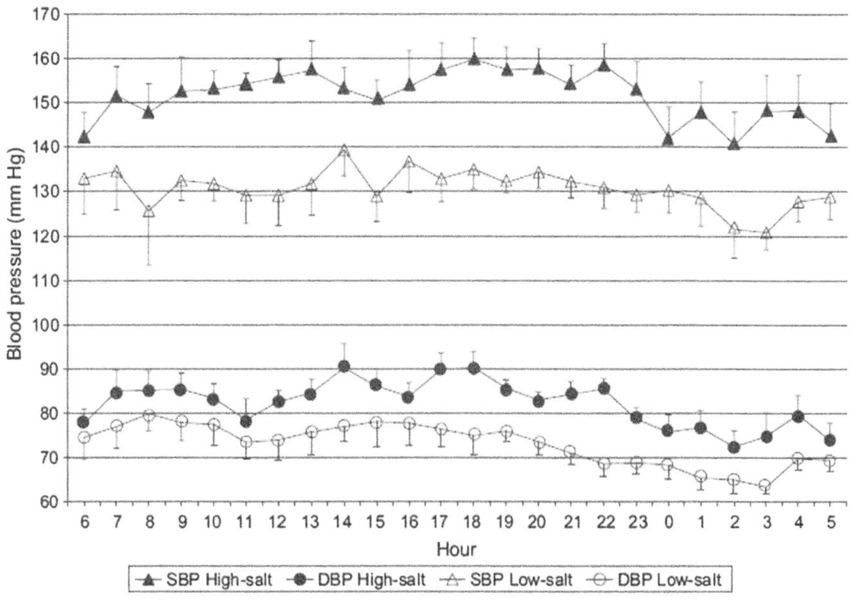

Fig. 7.2 Comparison of 24-hour ambulatory blood pressure values during low- and high-salt diet. The *low-salt meals* were formulated to provide 50 mmol of sodium per day (3 g/day). During high dietary salt intake, NaCl tablets (6 g/24 h) were added to the subject's regular diet with the intention to increase dietary sodium intake to >250 mmol/d (15 g/day). Data presented as mean ±SE. Figure from Pimenta et.al. [38]

In a recent study, patients were counseled to choose foods low in sodium and limit the amounts of added salt. A greater effect of sodium restriction was observed when a reduced salt intake is combined with other dietary counseling, for example in people who follow the Dietary Approaches to Stop Hypertension (DASH) diet or who have a high potassium intake [37, 39].

Data linking a decreased salt intake to a decrease in morbidity and mortality in hypertensive patients are not unanimous. Dietary salt intake reduction can delay or prevent the incidence of antihypertensive therapy and may represent a simple cost-saving mediator to reduce cardiovascular morbidity and mortality [37].
Question for the daily work: Does the patient limit dietary salt intake?
Therapeutic instrument: Recommend dietary sodium restriction per guidelines.

7.4.3 Alcohol

While modest consumption of alcohol (<30 g or 2 drinks/day) has not been associated with BP increases in most studies, heavy alcohol intake is associated with increased risk of hypertension [35]. A large intake of alcohol (>30 g) has a dose-related and biphasic effect on BP. It may lower BP in the first 4 h after ingestion, with BP elevation occurring approximately 10–15 h later. Heavy drinking is associated with a higher prevalence of HTN, hemorrhagic stroke, and cardiomyopathy [40], whereas moderate drinking is associated with lower prevalence of coronary artery disease, ischemic stroke, and sudden cardiac death [41, 42].

Patients should be counseled to reduce alcohol consumption to <2 drinks/day. Some recommendations counsel lower limits for women and lighter weight [18]. Of note, blood pressure control might more difficult to achieve in heavy drinkers due to poor adherence in antihypertensive therapy.
Question for the daily work: Is the patient a heavy alcohol drinker?
Therapeutic instrument: Recommend moderation of alcohol intake.

7.4.4 Obstructive Sleep Apnea Syndrome

Obstructive sleep apnea syndrome (OSA), which is defined as preserved and increased respiratory effort despite partial or complete occlusion of the upper airway, is a strong and independent risk factor for the presence of hypertension and cardiovascular diseases [43–46]. Around 30 % of adults with high blood pressure have obstructive sleep apnea, and the prevalence doubles for each 10-year increase in age in both sexes. Diastolic hypertension is the first to rise in subclinical obstructive sleep apnea [47]. Cross-sectional studies indicate that the severity of OSA is related to systolic and diastolic BPs and that hypertension occurring in individuals with OSA is more likely to be severe and resistant to treatment [48, 49]. The prevalence and severity were significantly higher in men than in women with resistant hypertension. In addition, it has been shown that OSA in normotensive subjects predicts future development of hypertension [35, 50].

A position paper published in 2012 on the management of patients with obstructive sleep apnea and hypertension recommends on the one hand lifestyle changes, like weight loss for decreasing the high blood pressure, and on the other hand also the therapy of antihypertensive drugs [50]. In an observational study, a weight loss of 10 % predicted a 26 % decrease in apnea hypopnea index. However, in only a few of these small-scale observational studies, information on BP changes was provided, and even massive weight loss and the reduction in OSA were found to result in proportionally modest and sometimes non-significant reductions in BP [35, 50].

Many studies have assessed the impact of active therapy of OSA on BP levels both in normotensive and in hypertensive patients with variable results [50]. Bazzano et al. [51] included in their meta-analysis 16 randomized clinical trials, with over 800 participants, who compared CPAP to control, had a minimum treatment duration of 2 weeks, and reported BP changes during the intervention or control period. Change in blood pressure for those treated with CPAP compared with control subject was −2.46 mm Hg/−1.83 mm Hg. In accordance, Alajmi et al. [52] conducted a literature search and identified 10 randomized, controlled trials with an appropriate control group. In this analysis with 587 patients, CPAP reduced blood pressure by 1.38/1.53 mm Hg [52]. These results demonstrated rather small effects, but individually justified changes, and control of BP may be observed. Aside from the small blood pressure–lowering effects, reduction in cardiovascular risk may occur nevertheless [50].

Screening test for obstructive sleep apnea: Questionnaire, overnight at-home sleep monitoring,

Findings: record cessations or reductions in airflow or chest wall movements of $\geq$10 s/h *of sleep and decrease in oxygen saturation.*

7.5 Non-adherence to Drug Therapy

Non-adherence is a major contributor to suboptimal medical treatment and results in uncontrolled hypertension. Common causes of non-adherence include lack of knowledge about hypertension, underestimation of the individual cardiovascular risk, effects of the antihypertensive medication, lack of efficacy and number of drugs, and pill and financial barriers in some conditions.

Thus, close follow-up visits addressing the non-compliance issue may improve adherence and persistence of antihypertensive medication. In long-term clinical trials, antihypertensive therapy discontinuation rates, were carefully assessed for different agents [53]. In this population-based cohort study with 109,454 patients, overall antihypertensive drug discontinuation was lower, with 20 % at 6 months and 30 % at 1 year. The median time to discontinuation was three years. 45 % who discontinue their first antihypertensive drug failed to switch to a different drug (or drug class) within three months of discontinuation [53]. It is important that general practitioners monitor patients closely in the first year following antihypertensive drug initiation, due to the high early risk of discontinuation. Non-adherence to drug therapy (even monotherapy) has been shown to increase hypertension-associated complications [54].

Because polypharmacy and complexity of blood pressure therapy regimen are known to be 2 of the determinants of poor medication compliance, efforts have been made to simplify the treatment regimen. Interventions aimed to simplify the drug regimen for patients (e.g., daily dosing as opposed to twice daily dosing) have been shown to improve patients' compliance in studies. Adherence evaluated by electronic monitoring falls from 79 % in patients taking medications once daily to 51 % with 4 times daily dosing [53]. Fixed-dose combinations are designed to simplify the medication regimen and potentially improve compliance. Bangalore analyzed data from studies with nearly 12.000 patients on fixed-dose combination versus 8300 patients on free-drug component regimen [55]. Fixed-dose combination resulted in a 26 % decrease in the risk of non-compliance compared with free-drug component regimen (Fig. 7.3). Fixed-dose combination therefore should be considered in patients with hypertension for improving medication compliance which can translate into better clinical outcomes. Even single-pill combinations of

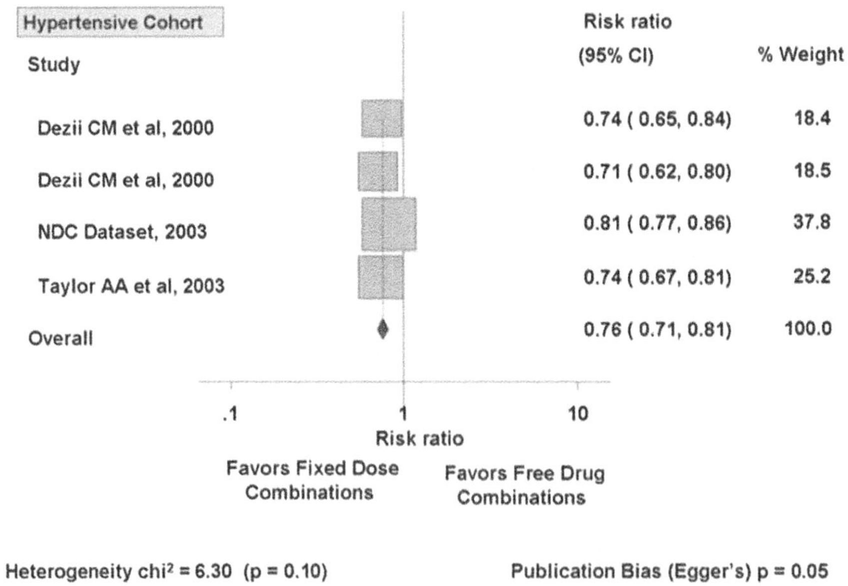

Fig. 7.3 Effect of fixed-dose combination versus free-drug combination on the risk of medication non-compliance in cohort with hypertension. *Vertical solid line* = null effect; *vertical dotted line* = overall effect on compliance; *boxes and horizontal lines* = relative risk (95 % CI). Figure from Bangalore et.al. [55]

≥3 antihypertensive agents became available in varying dosages [54], so most hypertensive patients can be controlled with fewer pills per day [56].

Another important aspect is that the chances of success of a long-term treatment of a chronic and generally asymptomatic disease such as hypertension remain tied to the patient–physician relationship. Barriers to implementation relate to both the clinician and the patient, and to their relationship. The degree of patient satisfaction at the end of a consultation is directly related to how the physician views the physician–patient relationship (patient-centered relationship and partnership between the two people, rather than a physician-controlled relationship) [57] and the involvement of patients regarding their care program. Such patient-centered relationship may have measurable effects on BP control [58]. A likely possibility, for explaining these results, is that physician's motivation could be a strong ingredient in motivating patients and supporting them to achieve a healthier lifestyle, leading to a better BP control, independently of clinical, therapeutic, sociodemographic, and behavioral characteristics of the patients themselves.

A controlled clinical trial [59] showed that physicians who were trained to educate patients could change their patients' behavior, making them more compliant, thus improving the likelihood of successfully controlling their BP. The 'highly motivated' physicians had a more confident approach to hypertension, looked more empathetic and supportive toward hypertensive patients, and exhibited an optimistic and rewarding patient–physician relationship [57, 59].

Question for the daily work: Does the patient adhere to the drug regimen?
Diagnostic instrument: Address patient adherence issues

7.6 Continuous Intake of Drug that Cause Hypertension

Several pharmacologic agents as well as some exogenous substances may induce hypertension. Drug-induced hypertension is one of the most common causes of secondary hypertension (see fig. 7.1) and is frequently encountered in clinical practice [60]. Nevertheless, despite the frequent occurrence of drug-induced hypertension, GPs frequently miss the opportunity to detect and manage this form of secondary hypertension. A detailed medical history in this field is of great importance in patients with resistant hypertension, because the identification and subsequent withdrawal of the drug may dissolve treatment resistance. In some cases, in which withdrawal of the responsible agent is not possible, dose reduction or search for alternate treatment may improve blood pressure levels.

7.6.1 Non-steroidal Anti-Inflammatory Drugs

The most common cause of drug-induced hypertension is the use of NSAIDs. In nearly 90 % of these cases, NSAIDs were being responsible [60]. Since osteoarthritis and hypertension often coexist (approximately half of the patients with osteoarthritis suffer from hypertension), the use of NSAIDs often causes resistant hypertension. Although the blood increase is on average 'only' 5–10 mmHg systolic and 2–5 mmHg diastolic, the individual response varies widely, with up to 50 mmHg increase in some individuals [61, 62].

This adverse effect has not significantly improved with the selective COX-2 inhibitors [63]. In a meta-analysis of randomized trials, use of COX-2 inhibitors was also associated with an increase in blood pressure compared to placebo and non-selective NSAIDs [64]. It was shown that a part of blood pressure elevation could be specifically attributed to rofecoxib [64], whereas other COX-2 inhibitors appeared to affect blood pressure to a lesser extent [63, 64]. The study showed another aspect, namely that there exist differences on blood pressure increases by the various NSAIDs. In a meta-analysis of randomized trials, naproxen and indomethacin were associated with the largest BP elevations, while piroxicam, sulindac, ibuprofen, and aspirin exhibited little or no effect on blood pressure (Fig. 7.4) [61].

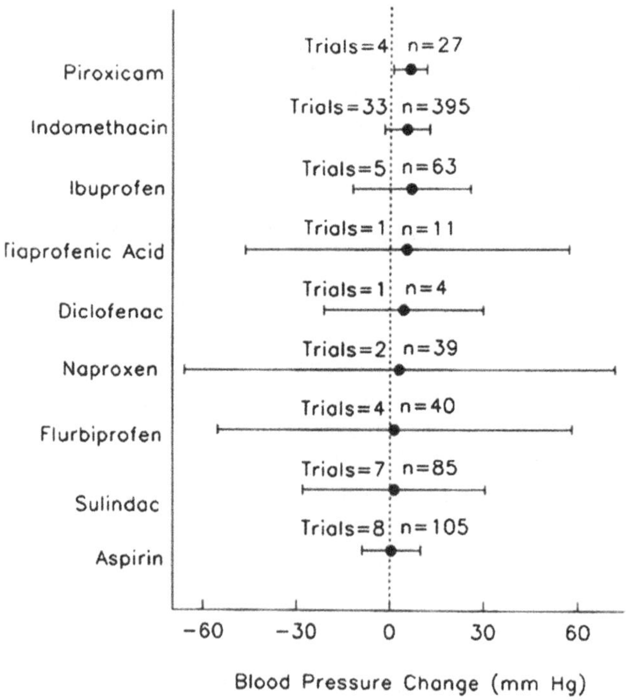

Fig. 7.4 A meta-analysis of randomized and placebo-controlled trials according to NSAID type and BP changes. A meta-analysis of randomized and placebo-controlled trials according to NSAID type showed that all NSAIDs increased supine mean blood pressure with piroxicam, indomethacin, and ibuprofen producing the most marked increases. Figure from Johnson et al. [61]

7.6.2 Corticosteroid

Oral glucocorticoids can increase systolic blood pressure as much as 15 mmHg within 24 h. Glucocorticoid-induced hypertension occurs more often in the elderly compared with younger patients [33]. Mineralocorticoids and other compounds, such as licorice and carbenoxolone, that inhibit the 11 beta-hydroxysteroid dehydrogenase enzyme, increase exchangeable sodium and blood volume, induce hyperkalemia and metabolic alkalosis, and suppress plasma renin activity.

7.6.3 Oral Contraceptives

Oral contraceptives are another class of drugs that may induce hypertension [65]. Oral contraceptives result on average in only a mild elevation of blood pressure but cause hypertension in approximately 5 % of users of high-dose pills. In prospective trials, current users of oral contraceptives had an increased risk (nearly twofold risk) of developing arterial hypertension compared to women who had never hypertension in about 5 %. This risk for past users was 20 % [65]. A big study that evaluates the effects of oral contraceptives on BP was the Nurses' Health Study, in which more than 60,000 normotensive women were prospectively followed for 4 years. Women using oral contraceptives had a higher risk of developing hypertension compared to women without consuming such medications [66].

The type of oral contraceptives also seems to be of clinical importance. Both estrogen and progestogen may be responsible for the BP effect, but the mechanism is as yet unknown. The combination of oral contraceptives (progestin and estradiol), which were widely used in the past, was more often associated with blood pressure elevations than progestin-only oral contraceptives. On the other side, drospirenone reduces blood pressure when combined with estradiol [67]. Oral contraceptives induce hypertension if high-dose pills are taken that contain at least 50 μg estrogen and 1–4 mg progestin [65]. Preparations with an estrogen content of 30 μg and a progestogen content of 1 mg or less seem to be without risk [68].

Postmenopausal oral estrogen therapy has been also discussed to induce hypertension. In a prospective placebo-controlled trials (222 healthy postmenopausal women), no significant blood pressure was observed on average [69]. However, a significant interaction with age was noted, indicating increase in systolic blood pressure in younger postmenopausal women, while having the opposite effect in older postmenopausal women [69].

7.6.4 Anti-VEGF Agents and Others

Antineoplastic drugs that target the VEGF pathway are another class of drugs that emerged as inducers of hypertension [70]. High blood pressure often was encountered in patients receiving VEGF inhibitors. 20–30 % of patients treated with bevacizumab, and up to 60 % of patients treated with VEGF kinase inhibitors developed hypertension [71]. Three meta-analyses with drugs inhibiting the VEGF pathway showed a high relative risk of incident hypertension with these agents: 7.5 with bevacizumab, 6.11 with sorafenib, and 21.6 with sunitinib [72].

Other important groups of drugs that can cause an increase in blood pressure are, for example, the sympathomimetics (diet pills, amphetamines), the antidepressants, and the erythropoietin agent and are listed in Fig. 7.1.

Question for the daily work: Does the patient take interfering substances?

Diagnostic instrument: Discontinue or minimize interfering or competing substances.

7.7 Conclusion

The etiology of resistant arterial hypertension is multifactorial: Numerous risk factors and comorbidities are associated with therapy resistance. In consequence, the key to managing resistant hypertension lies in a careful elicitation of the history, a meticulous examination of the patient, and good investigational backup, primarily to exclude secondary causes of hypertension. It should be emphasized that the patient's history may well provide the key to identify secondary causes of hypertension.

References

1. Calhoun DA, Jones D, Textor S, Goff DC, Murphy TP, Toto RD, White A, Cushman WC, White W, Sica D, Ferdinand K, Giles TD, Falkner B, Carey RM (2008) Resistant hypertension: diagnosis, evaluation, and treatment: a scientific statement from the American heart association professional education committee of the council for high blood pressure research. Circulation 117:e510–e526
2. Pimenta E, Calhoun DA (2012) Resistant hypertension: incidence, prevalence, and prognosis. Circulation 125:1594–1596
3. White WB, Maraka S (2012) Is it possible to manage hypertension and evaluate therapy without ambulatory blood pressure monitoring? Curr Hypertens Rep 14:366–373
4. Rasmussen SL, Torp-Pedersen C, Borch-Johnsen K, Ibsen H (1998) Normal values for ambulatory blood pressure and differences between casual blood pressure and ambulatory blood pressure: results from a Danish population survey. J Hypertens 16:1415–1424
5. Manios ED, Koroboki EA, Tsivgoulis GK, Spengos KM, Spiliopoulou IK, Brodie FG, Vemmos KN, Zakopoulos NA (2008) Factors influencing white-coat effect. Am J Hypertens 21:153–158
6. Messerli FH, Ventura HO, Amodeo C (1985) Osler's maneuver and pseudohypertension. N Engl J Med 312:1548–1551
7. Wright JC, Looney SW (1997) Prevalence of positive Osler's manoeuver in 3387 persons screened for the systolic hypertension in the elderly program (SHEP). J Hum Hypertens 11:285–289
8. Aronow WS, Fleg JL, Pepine CJ, Artinian NT, Bakris G, Brown AS, Ferdinand KC, Ann Forciea M, Frishman WH, Jaigobin C, Kostis JB, Mancia G, Oparil S, Ortiz E, Reisin E,

Rich MW, Schocken DD, Weber MA, Wesley DJ (2011) ACCF/AHA 2011 expert consensus document on hypertension in the elderly. J Am Coll Cardiol 2011(57):2037–2114
9. Spence JD (1997) Pseudo-hypertension in the elderly: still hazy, after all these years. J Hum Hypertens 11:621–623
10. Dworkin LD, Cooper CJ (2009) Clinical practice. Renal-artery stenosis. N Engl J Med 361:1972–1978
11. Safian RD, Textor SC (2001) Renal-artery stenosis. N Engl J Med 344:431–442
12. Textor SC (2002) Progressive hypertension in a patient with "incidental" renal artery stenosis. Hypertension 40:595–600
13. Garovic VD, Textor SC (2005) Renovascular hypertension and ischemic nephropathy. Circulation 112:1362–1374
14. McPhaul JJ Jr, McIntosh DA, Williams LF, Gritti EJ, Malette WG, Grollman A (1965) Remediable hypertension due to unilateral renal disease: correlation of split renal-function tests and pressor assays of renal venous blood in hypertensive patients. Arch Intern Med 115:644–651
15. Kirkendall WM, Fitz AE, Lawrence MS (1967) Renal hypertension. Diagnosis and surgical treatment. N Engl J Med 276:479–485
16. Birrer M, Do DD, Mahler F, Triller J, Baumgartner I (2002) Treatment of renal artery fibromuscular dysplasia with balloon angioplasty: a prospective follow-up study. Eur J Vasc Endovasc Surg 23:146–152
17. Alhadad A, Mattiasson I, Ivancev K, Gottsater A, Lindblad B (2005) Revascularisation of renal artery stenosis caused by fibromuscular dysplasia: effects on blood pressure during 7-year follow-up are influenced by duration of hypertension and branch artery stenosis. J Hum Hypertens 19:761–767
18. Mancia G, De Backer G, Dominiczak A, Cifkova R, Fagard R, Germano G, Grassi G, Heagerty AM, Kjeldsen SE, Laurent S, Narkiewicz K, Ruilope L, Rynkiewicz A, Schmieder RE, Boudier HA, Zanchetti A, Vahanian A, Camm J, De Caterina R, Dean V, Dickstein K, Filippatos G, Funck-Brentano C, Hellemans I, Kristensen SD, McGregor K, Sechtem U, Silber S, Tendera M, Widimsky P, Zamorano JL, Erdine S, Kiowski W, Agabiti-Rosei E, Ambrosioni E, Lindholm LH, Viigimaa M, Adamopoulos S, Bertomeu V, Clement D, Farsang C, Gaita D, Lip G, Mallion JM, Manolis AJ, Nilsson PM, O'Brien E, Ponikowski P, Redon J, Ruschitzka F, Tamargo J, van Zwieten P, Waeber B, Williams B (2007) Guidelines for the management of arterial hypertension (ESC). J Hypertens 25:1105–1187
19. Levey AS, Coresh J, Balk E, Kausz AT, Levin A, Steffes MW, Hogg RJ, Perrone RD, Lau J, Eknoyan G (2003) National kidney foundation practice guidelines for chronic kidney disease: evaluation, classification, and stratification. Ann Intern Med 139:137–147
20. Funder JW, Carey RM, Fardella C, Gomez-Sanchez CE, Mantero F, Stowasser M, Young WF Jr, Montori VM (2008) Case detection, diagnosis, and treatment of patients with primary aldosteronism: an endocrine society clinical practice guideline. J Clin Endocrinol Metab 93:3266–3281
21. Douma S, Petidis K, Doumas M et al (2008) Prevalence of primary hyperaldosteronism in resistant hypertension: a retrospective observational study. Lancet 371:1921–1926
22. Faselis C, Doumas M, Papademetriou V (2011) Common secondary causes of resistant hypertension and rational for treatment. Int J Hypertens 2011:236239
23. Calhoun DA, Nishizaka MK, Zaman MA, Thakkar RB, Weissmann P (2002) Hyperaldosteronism among black and white subjects with resistant hypertension. Hypertension 40:892–896
24. Stowasser M (2009) Update in primary aldosteronism. J Clin Endocrinol Metab 94:3623–3630
25. Mosso L, Carvajal C, Gonzalez A, Barraza A, Avila F, Montero J, Huete A, Gederlini A, Fardella CE (2003) Primary aldosteronism and hypertensive disease. Hypertension 42:161–165

26. Strauch B, Zelinka T, Hampf M, Bernhardt R, Widimsky J Jr (2003) Prevalence of primary hyperaldosteronism in moderate to severe hypertension in the Central Europe region. J Hum Hypertens 17:349–352
27. Tamura Y, Adachi J, Chiba Y, Mori S, Takeda K, Kasuya Y, Murayama T, Sawabe M, Sasano H, Araki A, Ito H, Horiuchi T (2008) Primary aldosteronism due to unilateral adrenal microadenoma in an elderly patient: efficacy of selective adrenal venous sampling. Intern Med 47:37–42
28. Stowasser M, Taylor PJ, Pimenta E, Ahmed AH, Gordon RD (2010) Laboratory investigation of primary aldosteronism. Clin Biochem Rev 31:39–56
29. Mulatero P, Rabbia F, Milan A, Paglieri C, Morello F, Chiandussi L, Veglio F (2002) Drug effects on aldosterone/plasma renin activity ratio in primary aldosteronism. Hypertension 40:897–902
30. Vonend O, Ockenfels N, Gao X, Allolio B, Lang K, Mai K, Quack I, Saleh A, Degenhart C, Seufert J, Seiler L, Beuschlein F, Quinkler M, Podrabsky P, Bidlingmaier M, Lorenz R, Reincke M, Rump LC (2011) Adrenal venous sampling: evaluation of the German conn's registry. Hypertension 57:990–995
31. Manger WM (2006) An overview of pheochromocytoma: history, current concepts, vagaries, and diagnostic challenges. Ann N Y Acad Sci 1073:1–20
32. Lenders JW, Eisenhofer G, Mannelli M, Pacak K (2005) Phaeochromocytoma. Lancet 366:665–675
33. Aronow WS, Fleg JL, Pepine CJ, Artinian NT, Bakris G, Brown AS, Ferdinand KC, Ann Forciea M, Frishman WH, Jaigobin C, Kostis JB, Mancia G, Oparil S, Ortiz E, Reisin E, Rich MW, Schocken DD, Weber MA, Wesley DJ (2011) ACCF/AHA 2011 expert consensus document on hypertension in the elderly: a report of the American college of cardiology foundation task force on clinical expert consensus documents developed in collaboration with the American academy of neurology, American geriatrics society, American society for preventive cardiology, American society of hypertension, American society of nephrology, Association of black cardiologists, and European society of hypertension. J Am Coll Cardiol 57:2037–2114
34. Streeten DH, Anderson GH Jr, Howland T, Chiang R, Smulyan H (1988) Effects of thyroid function on blood pressure. Recognition of hypothyroid hypertension. Hypertension 11:78–83
35. Frisoli TM, Schmieder RE, Grodzicki T, Messerli FH (2011) Beyond salt: lifestyle modifications and blood pressure. Eur Heart J 32:3081–3087
36. Appel LJ, Giles TD, Black HR, Izzo JL Jr, Materson BJ, Oparil S, Weber MA (2009) ASH position paper: dietary approaches to lower blood pressure. J Clin Hypertens (Greenwich) 11:358–368
37. Frisoli TM, Schmieder RE, Grodzicki T, Messerli FH (2012) Salt and hypertension: is salt dietary reduction worth the effort? Am J Med 125:433–439
38. Pimenta E, Gaddam KK, Oparil S, Aban I, Husain S, Dell'Italia LJ, Calhoun DA (2009) Effects of dietary sodium reduction on blood pressure in subjects with resistant hypertension: results from a randomized trial. Hypertension 54:475–481
39. Sacks FM, Svetkey LP, Vollmer WM, Appel LJ, Bray GA, Harsha D, Obarzanek E, Conlin PR, Miller ER 3rd, Simons-Morton DG, Karanja N, Lin PH (2001) Effects on blood pressure of reduced dietary sodium and the dietary approaches to stop hypertension (DASH) diet. DASH-sodium collaborative research group. N Engl J Med 344:3–10
40. Klatsky AL (2005) Alcohol and stroke: an epidemiological labyrinth. Stroke 36:1835–1836
41. Klatsky AL (2003) Drink to your health? Sci Am 288:74–81
42. Ronksley PE, Brien SE, Turner BJ, Mukamal KJ, Ghali WA (2011) Association of alcohol consumption with selected cardiovascular disease outcomes: a systematic review and meta-analysis. BMJ 342:d671
43. Peppard PE, Young T, Palta M, Skatrud J (2000) Prospective study of the association between sleep-disordered breathing and hypertension. N Engl J Med 342:1378–1384

44. Nieto FJ, Young TB, Lind BK, Shahar E, Samet JM, Redline S, D'Agostino RB, Newman AB, Lebowitz MD, Pickering TG (2000) Association of sleep-disordered breathing, sleep apnea, and hypertension in a large community-based study. Sleep heart health study. JAMA 283:1829–1836
45. Somers VK, White DP, Amin R, Abraham WT, Costa F, Culebras A, Daniels S, Floras JS, Hunt CE, Olson LJ, Pickering TG, Russell R, Woo M, Young T (2008) Sleep apnea and cardiovascular disease: an American heart association/american college of cardiology foundation scientific statement from the American heart association council for high blood pressure research professional education committee, council on clinical cardiology, stroke council, and council on cardiovascular nursing. In collaboration with the national heart, lung, and blood institute national center on sleep disorders research (National Institutes of Health). Circulation 118:1080–1111
46. Somers VK, White DP, Amin R, Abraham WT, Costa F, Culebras A, Daniels S, Floras JS, Hunt CE, Olson LJ, Pickering TG, Russell R, Woo M, Young T (2008) Sleep apnea and cardiovascular disease: an American heart association/american college of cardiology foundation scientific statement from the American heart association council for high blood pressure research professional education committee, council on clinical cardiology, stroke council, and council on cardiovascular nursing. J Am Coll Cardiol 52:686–717
47. Sharabi Y, Scope A, Chorney N, Grotto I, Dagan Y (2003) Diastolic blood pressure is the first to rise in association with early subclinical obstructive sleep apnea: lessons from periodic examination screening. Am J Hypertens 16:236–239
48. Grote L, Ploch T, Heitmann J, Knaack L, Penzel T, Peter JH (1999) Sleep-related breathing disorder is an independent risk factor for systemic hypertension. Am J Respir Crit Care Med 160:1875–1882
49. Calhoun DA, Harding SM (2010) Sleep and hypertension. Chest 138:434–443
50. Parati G, Lombardi C, Hedner J, Bonsignore MR, Grote L, Tkacova R, Levy P, Riha R, Bassetti C, Narkiewicz K, Mancia G, McNicholas WT (2012) Position paper on the management of patients with obstructive sleep apnea and hypertension: joint recommendations by the European society of hypertension, by the european respiratory society and by the members of European COST (CO-operation in scientific and technological research) ACTION B26 on obstructive sleep apnea. J Hypertens 30:633–646
51. Bazzano LA, Khan Z, Reynolds K, He J (2007) Effect of nocturnal nasal continuous positive airway pressure on blood pressure in obstructive sleep apnea. Hypertension 50:417–423
52. Alajmi M, Mulgrew AT, Fox J, Davidson W, Schulzer M, Mak E, Ryan CF, Fleetham J, Choi P, Ayas NT (2007) Impact of continuous positive airway pressure therapy on blood pressure in patients with obstructive sleep apnea hypopnea: a meta-analysis of randomized controlled trials. Lung 185:67–72
53. Burke TA, Sturkenboom MC, Lu SE, Wentworth CE, Lin Y, Rhoads GG (2006) Discontinuation of antihypertensive drugs among newly diagnosed hypertensive patients in UK general practice. J Hypertens 24:1193–1200
54. Mathes J, Kostev K, Gabriel A, Pirk O, Schmieder RE (2010) Relation of the first hypertension-associated event with medication, compliance and persistence in naive hypertensive patients after initiating monotherapy. Int J Clin Pharmacol Ther 48:173–183
55. Bangalore S, Kamalakkannan G, Parkar S, Messerli FH (2007) Fixed-dose combinations improve medication compliance: a meta-analysis. Am J Med 120:713–719
56. Black HR (2009) Triple fixed-dose combination therapy: back to the past. Hypertension 54:19–22
57. Consoli SM, Lemogne C, Levy A, Pouchain D, Laurent S (2010) Physicians' degree of motivation regarding their perception of hypertension, and blood pressure control. J Hypertens 28:1330–1339
58. Orth JE, Stiles WB, Scherwitz L, Hennrikus D, Vallbona C (1987) Patient exposition and provider explanation in routine interviews and hypertensive patients' blood pressure control. Health Psychol 6:29–42

59. Inui TS, Yourtee EL, Williamson JW (1976) Improved outcomes in hypertension after physician tutorials. A controlled trial. Ann Intern Med 84:646–651
60. Forman JP, Rimm EB, Curhan GC (2007) Frequency of analgesic use and risk of hypertension among men. Arch Intern Med 167:394–399
61. Johnson AG, Nguyen TV, Day RO (1994) Do nonsteroidal anti-inflammatory drugs affect blood pressure? A meta-analysis. Ann Intern Med 121:289–300
62. Pope JE, Anderson JJ, Felson DT (1993) A meta-analysis of the effects of nonsteroidal anti-inflammatory drugs on blood pressure. Arch Intern Med 153:477–484
63. White WB, Kent J, Taylor A, Verburg KM, Lefkowith JB, Whelton A (2002) Effects of celecoxib on ambulatory blood pressure in hypertensive patients on ACE inhibitors. Hypertension 39:929–934
64. Wolfe F, Zhao S, Pettitt D (2004) Blood pressure destabilization and edema among 8538 users of celecoxib, rofecoxib, and nonselective nonsteroidal antiinflammatory drugs (NSAID) and nonusers of NSAID receiving ordinary clinical care. J Rheumatol 31:1143–1151
65. Chasan-Taber L, Willett WC, Manson JE, Spiegelman D, Hunter DJ, Curhan G, Colditz GA, Stampfer MJ (1996) Prospective study of oral contraceptives and hypertension among women in the United States. Circulation 94:483–489
66. Lubianca JN, Faccin CS, Fuchs FD (2003) Oral contraceptives: a risk factor for uncontrolled blood pressure among hypertensive women. Contraception 67:19–24
67. White WB, Hanes V, Chauhan V, Pitt B (2006) Effects of a new hormone therapy, drospirenone and 17-beta-estradiol, in postmenopausal women with hypertension. Hypertension 48:246–253
68. Woods JW (1988) Oral contraceptives and hypertension. Hypertension 11:II11–II15
69. Steiner AZ, Hodis HN, Lobo RA, Shoupe D, Xiang M, Mack WJ (2005) Postmenopausal oral Estrogen therapy and blood pressure in normotensive and hypertensive subjects: the Estrogen in the prevention of atherosclerosis trial. Menopause 12:728–733
70. Hurwitz H, Fehrenbacher L, Novotny W, Cartwright T, Hainsworth J, Heim W, Berlin J, Baron A, Griffing S, Holmgren E, Ferrara N, Fyfe G, Rogers B, Ross R, Kabbinavar F (2004) Bevacizumab plus irinotecan, fluorouracil, and leucovorin for metastatic colorectal cancer. N Engl J Med 350:2335–2342
71. Verheul HM, Pinedo HM (2007) Possible molecular mechanisms involved in the toxicity of angiogenesis inhibition. Nat Rev Cancer 7:475–485
72. Wu S, Chen JJ, Kudelka A, Lu J, Zhu X (2008) Incidence and risk of hypertension with sorafenib in patients with cancer: a systematic review and meta-analysis. Lancet Oncol 9:117–123

24-hour Ambulatory BP Monitoring and Home BP Measurements in Resistant Hypertension

8

Josep Redon and Fernando Martinez

8.1 Introduction

Hypertensive patients whose clinic blood pressure (BP) remains persistently high despite taking three or more antihypertensive drugs are defined as having resistant hypertension and account for 10 % of hypertensive subjects referred to specialized clinics [1–4]. zDespite extensive diagnostic work-up, in many cases, it is not possible to find a potentially correctable cause of the elevated BP, even though compliance to medication seems to be adequate [5–7]. Patients whose hypertension is uncontrolled are more likely to have target organ damage and a higher long-term cardiovascular risk than are patients whose BP is controlled. The definition, prevalence, and incidence vary according to the origin of the data, but today, it is accepted to define resistant hypertension if BP is ≥140/90 mmHg in antihypertensive medications with 3 different drug classes or drugs from ≥4 antihypertensive drug classes regardless of BP. Among US adults with hypertension, 8.9 % met criteria for resistant hypertension in a recent report from NHANES [8]. Among patients with incident hypertension in whom treatment was begun, 1 in 50 patients developed resistant hypertension [9] and they have an increased risk of cardiovascular events, which supports the need for greater efforts to reduce hypertension outcomes. The relative high prevalence of resistant hypertension in the office is drastically reduced when potential confounding factors are ruled-out. Regression to the mean of BP values when measurements are repeated, low adherence to antihypertensive treatment [10] and some common forms of secondary hypertension

J. Redon (✉) · F. Martinez
Hypertension Clinic, Internal Medicine, Hospital Clinico of Valencia, Research Institute, INCLIVA, University of Valencia, Avda Blasco Ibañez, 17, 46010 Valencia, Spain
e-mail: josep.redon@uv.es

J. Redon
CIBEROBN, Institute of Health Carlos III, Madrid, Spain

G. Mancia (ed.), *Resistant Hypertension*, DOI: 10.1007/978-88-470-5415-8_8,

such as sleep apnea and primary aldosteronism are frequent confounding factors [11]. The most frequent confounding factor, however, is the persistence of alarm reaction, the so-called white-coat reaction.

Since the persistence of "white-coat" reaction is frequent among patients uncontrolled during antihypertensive treatment, out-of-office BP measurements play an important role in the evaluation of resistant hypertension. In a large Spanish registry, about one-third of 8,295 patients with resistant hypertension based on office BP measurements had normal ABPM suggesting the presence of white-coat resistance [12]. In fact, 24 h ambulatory BP monitoring (ABPM) has been considered mandatory at the time to evaluate resistant hypertension from the beginning of clinical use. Furthermore, clinical research has expanded the potential role of out-of-office measurements not only to the initial evaluation of resistant hypertension but also to refine cardiovascular and renal risk stratification and for a better follow-up. Likewise, the widespread use of self-BP measurement at home (HBPM) [13] introduced a new tool to properly assess out-of-office BP and it has also been recommended in these patients although the potential differences between the two methods remain controversial.

8.2 ABPM in the Diagnosis

The recommendation to use out-of-office BP measurements in resistant hypertension is based on the evidence that ABPM gives better prognostic information than office measurement [14–16]. Three studies have demonstrated that higher baseline ambulatory systolic or diastolic BP predicts cardiovascular events better than office BP does. The first study showed that in patients with resistant hypertension, with or without a previous cardiovascular disease, ABPM was an independent marker of risk for new cardiovascular events, suggesting that ABPM was useful in stratifying the risk in patients with resistant hypertension [14]. Two additional studies [15, 16] have confirmed these results and reinforced the superiority of ABPM over office BP for stratifying risk (Table 8.1). The largest study was published by Selles et al. [16] with 556 subjects (average BP 178/99 mmHg) followed during an average of 57 months of whom 109 developed events. After adjustment for office BP, higher mean ambulatory BPs were independent predictors of the composite end point. The hazard ratios associated with a 1-SD

Table 8.1 Studies of prognostic value of ambulatory BP in resistant hypertension

Author, yr (ref)	Office SBP/DBP mmHg	Follow-up (months)	Patients	Events
Redon 1998 [14]	177/106	49	86	12
Pierdomenico 2005 [15]	162/95	60	270	46
Salles 2008 [16]	178/99	57	556	109
Redon 2009 [19]	172/96	56	386	32

increment in daytime and nighttime systolic BP were 1.26 (95 % CI, 1.04–1.53) and 1.38 (1.13–1.68), respectively; the corresponding values for diastolic BP were 1.31 (1.05–1.63) and 1.36 (1.10–1.69). Ambulatory systolic and diastolic BPs were equivalent predictors and both were better than pulse pressure [16].

All the studies on prognosis of ambulatory BP were carried out using only one monitoring at the beginning of the observational period [14–16]. The potential impact of BP changes over time, spontaneous or induced by antihypertensive treatment, has never been taken into account and seems to be clinically relevant. The importance of repeated BP measurements in prognosis has only been considered in two studies with ABPM, one in which the risk to develop microalbuminuria was associated with nocturnal BP in normotensive type 1 diabetes [17] and another in which the preservation of renal function was associated with effective reduction in ambulatory BP values [18]. In our group, a cohort of 386 subjects with initial BP 172/96 mmHg suffered 32 cardiovascular events during an average of 56 months. In this cohort, average of 24 h SBP >135 mmHg, the risk doubled as compared to those with values below 135 mmHg in a time-varied Cox regression analysis [19].

Beside the role of ABPM at the time to detect "white-coat," ABPM may also identify "masked" resistant hypertension in patients on multiple drug therapy who might have low office but elevated ambulatory BP [20]. This is particularly relevant in patients with chronic kidney disease (CKD). High BP is frequent in individuals with CKD and prevalence increases with declining glomerular filtration rate (GFR), so much so that up to 95 % of individuals with a GFR <15 ml/min are hypertensive [21, 22]. In patients with CKD, including those with functioning renal transplants, there are frequently not only high BP values, but also a blunting or loss of the normal physiological drop in BP measured at night [23–25] in a recent study from our group [26], which included 86 patients with CKD stage 3–4 with resistant hypertension, 63 % of the patients had office SBP >140 mmHg and 46 % of the patients had office DBP >90 mmHg, 86 % of the patients had 24 h systolic ABP and the same percentage had 24 h diastolic ABP (Fig. 8.1). Then, ABPM also uncovered an elevated percentage of patients with masked phenomenon, controlled in BP measured in office and uncontrolled 24 h ABP. The blunted physiological decline of BP at night can explain the high prevalence of masked phenomenon.

8.3 ABPM to Refine Risk Stratification

Although the most important prognostic factor in patients with resistant hypertension is the average of 24 h BP values, other parameters obtained with ABPM have demonstrated additional prognostic information above and beyond the average of 24 h BP values, mainly alteration of circadian variability and the ambulatory arterial stiffness index (AASI).

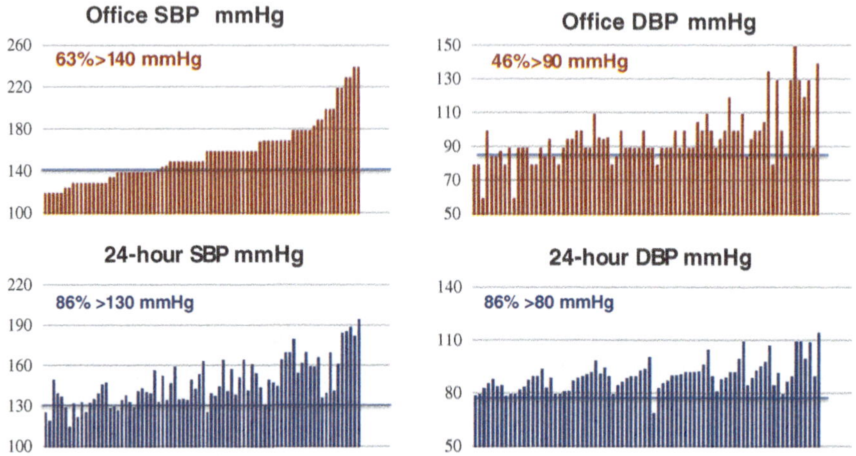

Fig. 8.1 Blood pressure values of chronic kidney disease stage 3–4 patients. Distribution of office systolic and diastolic BP and percentage of subjects with BP <140/90 mmHg (*upper graphs*). Distribution of 24 h ambulatory systolic and diastolic BP and percentage of subjects with BP <130/80 mmHg (*lower graphs*)

The prognostic value of nocturnal BP is particularly relevant. Muxfeldt et al. [27] published that the prevalence of non-dipping pattern was 65.0 %. After adjustment for several confounders, the non-dipping pattern was an independent predictor of cardiovascular events (HR 1.74; 95 % CI 1.12–2.71) and of cardiovascular mortality (HR, 2.31; 95 % CI, 1.09–4.92). The effect of the non-dipping pattern on cardiovascular prognosis was stronger in younger patients and in those with true resistant hypertension. This points to the importance of nocturnal BP values as a prognostic factor.

In 79 patients with CKD, the eGFR at entry to the study was a strong predictor, with a 1 ml/min reduction in eGFR increasing the risk of ESRD or death by 7 %. In a multivariate analysis that included age, sex, RAS blockade, and the three specified tertiles of eGFR, office BP measurements did not provide prognostic information on risk of ESRD or death [26]. Furthermore, daytime ambulatory SBP measurements (third tertile SBP >140 mmHg versus first tertile SBP <125 mmHg, HR 1.40, 95 % CI 0.63–3.14) and the dipper/non-dipper status (HR 0.92, 95 % CI 0.48–1.76) did not further discriminate in terms of predicting endpoint risk. Nocturnal SBP measurement in this model, however, provided relevant information. The third tertile of nocturnal SBP, >130 mmHg, was associated with a doubling of risk, HR 2.07 (95 % CI 1.01–4.25) of ESRD or of death, when compared to the risk associated with a nocturnal SBP <120 mmHg ($p = 0.047$) on top of the other significant factors (Fig. 8.2). The addition of daytime SBP did not remove systolic nocturnal BP from the model. Likewise, the risk of cardiovascular events, myocardial infarction, angina, congestive heart failure, or cardiovascular death, was also linked to the nocturnal SBP >129 mmHg increasing the risk by 3.6 times (95 % CI 1.2–9.2), Fig. 8.3 (*data unpublished*).

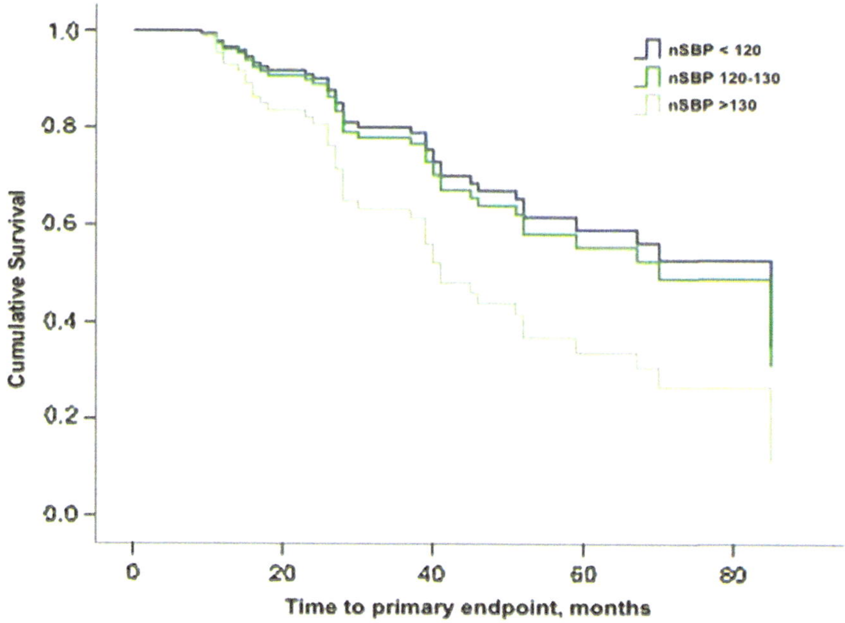

Fig. 8.2 Prognostic value of night SBP to develop ESRD or death in CKD stage 3–4 [26]

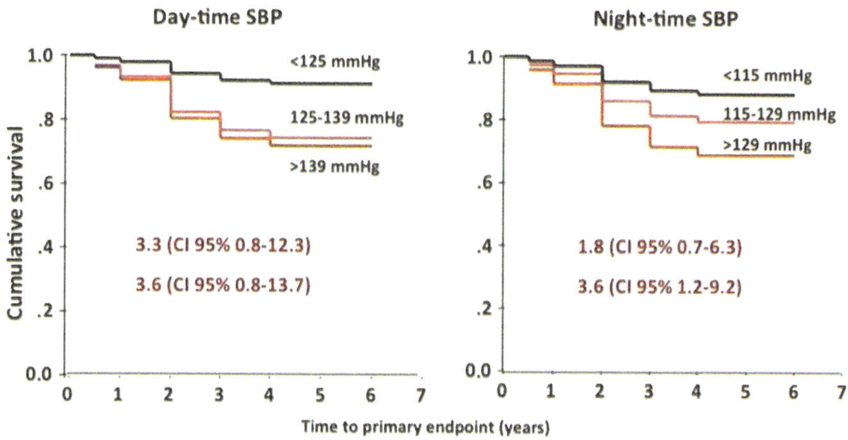

Fig. 8.3 Risk of cardiovascular outcomes (IMA, angina, CHF, CV death) according to the ambulatory SBP, independent of age, sex, Hb, and LVH. BP values are the average of the two monitorings during the follow-up

The fact that it is the nocturnal BP and not the non-dipping pattern which offered prognostic information in this population of CKD patient merits a general comment. The strongest relationship of nocturnal BP with progression of renal damage was previously described by our group [17] and others [28–31]. Although high nocturnal BP is sometimes accompanied by a non-dipping pattern, both are not always present together and its significance differs. Maintaining high BP at night overloads the kidney since it is during the resting period when the afferent arteriolar tone is lowest, allowing for a more direct transmission of the systemic BP to the glomerulus [32]. Consequently, high BP at night not only impacts the heart and the vasculature [33], but it also affects the kidney [32], boosting damage and increasing risk for developing clinical events. In contrast, the non-dipping pattern reflects inadequacy of the mechanisms regulating BP, and when a non-dipper pattern is present, it indicates a more advanced stage of organ damage as compared with subjects who maintain the physiological BP fall at night [34]. Therefore, in order to protect against progression of organ damage, nocturnal BP should be targeted regardless of the level of dipping.

The prognostic value of the AASI has also been investigated in resistant hypertension. This index, that is an indirect marker of arterial stiffness, resulted of prognostic value. 24 h AASI was the best independent predictor of cardiovascular events (HR 1.46, 95 % CI 1.12–1.92), whereas cardiovascular mortality was best predicted by nighttime AASI (HR 1.73, 95 % CI 1.13–2.65), after adjustments. 24 h AASI was a better predictor of cardiovascular outcomes in women, in younger and in non-diabetic individuals [35].

8.4 ABPM Uncovers Secondary Hypertension

Diagnosis of resistant hypertension requires the ruling-out of the presence of secondary hypertension by definition. Among the most frequent causes of secondary hypertension that call for a specific search, due to the frequent absence of specific clinical data, are primary aldosteronism and sleep apnea syndrome. In a recent study, among consecutive patients with resistant hypertension, obstructive sleep apnea appears to be the most common condition associated with resistant hypertension [11]. Likewise, primary aldosteronism was found in around 15 % of resistant hypertension in different series [36]. Non-dipping pattern is more common among both primary aldosteronism and sleep apnea syndrome in which an increase in aldosterone or adrenal hormones has been described. In fact, in a recent study of resistant hypertension, hypercortisolism was detected in a large percentage of subjects. In those with confirmed hypercortisolism with functional tests, the prevalence of non-dipping pattern was 77 % as compared with lower values in subjects without hypercortisolism [37]. It is possible that in patients with persistent non-dipping pattern it may be mandatory to exclude primary aldosteronism or sleep apnea syndrome. Furthermore, whether or not non-dipping pattern can be a marker of future response to antialdosterone drugs, is relevant clinical information. Up to now, only one study [38] analyzed the utility of several markers, such as K+, aldosterone, renin plasma activity, or the ratio aldosterone/plasma renin activity, in order to identify subjects that will respond better to antialdosterone drugs in resistant hypertension. Renin plasma activity and the ratio were significantly associated to SBP and DBP reduction, while K+ and aldosterone levels were not associated to the response.

Finally, the possibility to detect sharp BP elevation in the presence of pheochromocytoma [39] should be mentioned although the prevalence is very low and the possibility to capture BP peaks is even lower.

8.5 ABPM During the Follow-Up

If the measurement of office and ambulatory BP is important at the time to evaluate patients with resistant hypertension, assessment of BP during the follow-up is also a key issue. From the few observations available, discrepancies in the trends of office and ambulatory BP during the follow-up were observed. The change in BP during follow-up was analyzed by our group repeating the monitoring in 120 patients every second year. While office BP was reduced between the first and the second examinations, no additional reduction was observed later. This pattern was in contrast with the ambulatory BP which had continuously reducing BP values, mainly in diastolic and during the nighttime [19].

The discrepancies in the trend between office and ambulatory BP during the study can be explained by the persistence of the white-coat effect on office BP measurements coupled with the real impact of the treatment changes on ambulatory BP. The fact that in ambulatory BP the extent of BP reduction was higher in diastolic BP and during resting conditions as compared with the systolic and during activity argues that ambulatory BP is more influenced by antihypertensive treatment in this group of patients. Since changes were attributed in part to the effect of the antihypertensive treatment, reproducibility was not reported. It is noteworthy to acknowledge that in resistant hypertension, the "white-coat" phenomenon persists and even increases, driven by the additional impact of antihypertensive treatment.

In contrast, a recent study introduced a word of caution in the opposite sense, the reproducibility of "white-coat" phenomenon. In a prospective study which enrolled patients diagnosed as white-coat resistant hypertension on ABPM [40], a second confirmatory examination 3 months later and repeated twice at 6 month intervals was performed. When white-coat resistant hypertension diagnosis was remonitored after 3 months, it is still present in 144 from the initial 198 patients. In the third and fourth ABPMs, 74 and 79 % of patients sustained the diagnosis. The authors conclude that a confirmatory ABPM is necessary after 3 months of the first white-coat-resistant hypertension diagnosis, and the procedure should be repeated at 6 month intervals.

The high degree of variability among the BPs obtained during the study and the different trend observed for office and ambulatory BPs points to the necessity to monitor out-of-office BP during the follow-up of these very high-risk patients. Then, to assess BP control, out-of-office ABPM is mandatory, not only to check the success in the average of 24 h but also to ensure that the BP control is maintained across the most critical periods, nighttime, and even during the early morning surge.

Recent introduction of renal denervation (RDN) opens a new dimension in the therapeutic approach to resistant hypertension. RDN is a percutaneous procedure, minimally invasive, characterized by short recovery times, and absence of significant systematic side effects. Evidence on the clinical effectiveness of this procedure in hypertensive patients comes from the Simplicity Clinical Trial Program consisting of a group of studies focusing on the effects of RDN in the treatment of resistant hypertension. These trials include the Symplicity HTN-1 (with extended follow-up) and the Symplicity HTN-2 study, both already published [41–43].

Preliminary observations raised the doubt about the real efficacy of BP reduction after the procedure. In fact, the ratio between the SBP reduction in ambulatory and office in trials which have used antihypertensive drugs is around 80 %, while after RDN the ratio was around 30 % [44]. This can indicate that the beneficial BP lowering effect is limited to the sympathetic arousal and not during the 24 h. A similar low BP reduction during the 24 h was observed in sleep apnea syndrome, a situation in which sympathetic overactivity is underlying the BP elevation [45, 46]. More studies are necessary to clarify this important issue.

8.6 Self-BP Measurements

Self-BP measurement at home (HBPM) is a valuable method to assess out-of office BP with a good reproducibility, and in several consensus about its clinical utility, assessment of resistant hypertension was one of the common conditions [6, 7, 13]. Based on information obtained in another subgroup of hypertensives, HBPM can provide an estimation of BP close to the average of ABPM values. Then, HBPM can be helpful in the follow-up of these patients combined with the 24 h ABPM. However, in resistant hypertension, clinical ground information is scarce and a few studies have used it to diagnose true resistant hypertension. Marui et al. [47] compared the information obtained with ABPM and HBPM in a group of 51 patients with refractory hypertension. The comparison of mean daytime ABPM with HBPM average showed a good correlation for both systolic and diastolic BP values. True resistant hypertension was confirmed in 33 patients by ABPM and in 37 by HBPM. Similar results were obtained in 73 subjects published by Nasothimiou et al. [48]. HBPM was also used in some studies to diagnose true resistant hypertension such as in the Japan Home versus Office BP Measurement Evaluation, the J-HOME study [3]. In contrast to 24 h ABPM, HBPM do not permit assessment of BP at night as a valuable parameter as commented above. Likewise, no studies with prognostic information have been published to date in resistant hypertension.

References

1. Calhoun DA, Jones D, Textor S, American Heart Association Professional Education Committee et al (2008) Resistant hypertension: diagnosis, evaluation, and treatment: a scientific statement from the American Heart Association Professional Education Committee of the Council for High Blood Pressure Research. Circulation 117:e510–e526
2. Moser M, Setaro JF (2006) Resistant or difficult-to-control hypertension. N Engl J Med 355:385–392
3. Oikawa T, Obara T, Ohkubo T, J-HOME Study Group et al (2006) Characteristics of resistant hypertension determined by self-measured blood pressure at home and office blood pressure measurements: the J-HOME study. J Hypertens 24:1737–1743
4. Parker MG (2008) Resistant hypertension: core curriculum 2008. Am J Kidney Dis 52:796–802
5. Bunker J, Callister W, Chang CL et al (2011) How common is true resistant hypertension? J Hum Hypertens 25:137–140
6. Mancia G, de Backer G, Dominiczak A, Management of Arterial Hypertension of the European Society of Hypertension, European Society of Cardiology et al (2007) Guidelines for the Management of Arterial Hypertension: The Task Force for the Management of Arterial Hypertension of the European Society of Hypertension (ESH) and of the European Society of Cardiology (ESC). J Hypertens 25:1105–1187
7. Chobanian AV, Bakris GL, Black HR, Joint National Committee on Prevention, Detection, Evaluation, and Treatment of High Blood Pressure, National Heart, Lung, and Blood Institute, National High Blood Pressure Education Program Coordinating Committee et al (2003) Seventh report of the joint national committee on prevention, detection, evaluation, and treatment of high blood pressure. Hypertension 42(6):1206–1252
8. Persell SD (2011) Prevalence of resistant hypertension in the United States, 2003–2008. Hypertension 57:1076–1080
9. Daugherty SL, Powers JD, Magid DJ et al (2012) Incidence and prognosis of resistant hypertension in hypertensive patients. Circulation 125:1635–1642
10. Massierer D, Oliveira AC, Steinhorst AM et al (2012) Prevalence of resistant hypertension in non-elderly adults: prospective study in a clinical setting. Arq Bras Cardiol 99:630–635
11. Pedrosa RP, Drager LF, Gonzaga CC et al (2011) Obstructive sleep apnea: the most common secondary cause of hypertension associated with resistant hypertension. Hypertension 58:811–817
12. de la Sierra A, Segura J, Banegas JR et al (2011) Clinical features of 8,295 patients with resistant hypertension classified on the basis of ambulatory blood pressure monitoring. Hypertension 57:898–902
13. Parati G, Stergiou GS, Asmar R, ESH Working Group on Blood Pressure Monitoring et al (2008) European society of hypertension guidelines for blood pressure monitoring at home: a summary report of the second international consensus conference on home blood pressure monitoring. J Hypertens 26:1505–1526
14. Redon J, Campos C, Narciso ML et al (1998) Prognostic value of ambulatory blood pressure monitoring in refractory hypertension: a prospective study. Hypertension 31:712–718
15. Pierdomenico SD, Lapenna D, Bucci A et al (2005) Cardiovascular outcome in treated hypertensive patients with responder, masked, false resistant, and true resistant hypertension. Am J Hypertens 18:1422–1428
16. Salles GF, Cardoso CR, Muxfeldt ES (2008) Prognostic influence of office and ambulatory blood pressures in resistant hypertension. Arch Intern Med 168:2340–2346
17. Lurbe E, Redon J, Kesani A et al (2002) Increase in nocturnal blood pressure and progression to microalbuminuria in type 1 diabetes. N Engl J Med 347:797–805
18. ESCAPE Trial Group, Wühl E, Trivelli A, Picca S et al (2009) Strict blood-pressure control and progression of renal failure in children. N Engl J Med 361:1639–1650

19. Redon J, Oltra R, Rodilla E et al (2001) Prognostic value of repeated ambulatory blood pressure monitoring in refractory hypertension. J Clin Hypertens 13(suppl 1):134–135
20. Shafi S, Sarac E, Tran H (2012) Ambulatory blood pressure monitoring in patients with chronic kidney disease and resistant hypertension. J Clin Hypertens (Greenwich) 14:611–617
21. Parikh NI, Hwang SJ, Larson MG et al (2006) Cardiovascular disease risk factors in chronic kidney disease: overall burden and rates of treatment and control. Arch Intern Med 166:1884–1891
22. Buckalew VM, Berg RL, Wang SR et al (1996) Prevalence of hypertension in 1,795 subjects with chronic renal disease: the modification of diet in renal disease study baseline cohort. Modification of diet in renal disease study group. Am J Kidney Dis 28:811–821
23. Fukuda M, Munemura M, Usami T et al (2004) Nocturnal blood pressure is elevated with natriuresis and proteinuria as renal function deteriorated in nephropathy. Kidney Int 65:621–625
24. Farmer CK, Goldsmith DJ, Cox J et al (1997) An investigation of the effect of advancing uraemia, renal replacement therapy and renal transplantation on blood pressure diurnal variability. Nephrol Dial Transplant 12:2301–2307
25. Lurbe E, Redon J (1999) Assessing ambulatory blood pressure in renal diseases: facts and concerns. Nephrol Dial Transplant 14:2564–2568
26. Redon J, Plancha E, Swift PA et al (2010) Nocturnal blood pressure and progression to end-stage renal disease or death in nondiabetic chronic kidney disease stages 3 and 4. J Hypertens 28:602–607
27. Muxfeldt ES, Cardoso CR, Salles GF (2009) Prognostic value of nocturnal blood pressure reduction in resistant hypertension. Arch Intern Med 169:874–880
28. Csiky B, Kovaks T, Wagner L et al (1999) Ambulatory blood pressure monitoring and progression in patients with IgA nephropathy. Nephrol Dial Transplant 14:86–90
29. Timio M, Venanzi S, Lolli S et al (1995) "Non-dipper" hypertensive patients and progressive renal insufficiency: a 3-year longitudinal study. Clin Nephrol 43:382–387
30. Davidson MB, Hix JX, Vidt DG et al (2006) Association of impaired diurnal blood pressure variation with a subsequent decline in glomerular filtration rate. Arch Intern Med 166:846–852
31. Nakano S, Ogihara M, Tamura C et al (1999) Reversed circadian blood pressure rhythm independently predicts endstage renal failure in non–insulin-dependent diabetes mellitus subjects. J Diabetes Complications 13:224–231
32. Redon J, Lurbe E (2002) Ambulatory blood pressure and the kidney: implications for renal dysfunction. In: Epstein M (ed) Calcium antagonists in clinical medicine. Hanley & Belfus, Philadelphia, pp 665–679
33. Fagard RH, Celis H, Thijs L et al (2008) Daytime and nighttime blood pressure as predictors of death and cause-specific cardiovascular events in hypertension. Hypertension 51:55–61
34. Agarwal R, Light RP (2009) GFR, proteinuria and circadian blood pressure. Nephrol Dial Transplant 24:2400–2406
35. Muxfeldt ES, Cardoso CR, Dias VB et al (2010) Prognostic impact of the ambulatory arterial stiffness index in resistant hypertension. J Hypertens 28:1547–1553
36. Clark D 3rd, Ahmed MI, Calhoun DA (2012) Resistant hypertension and aldosterone: an update. Can J Cardiol 28:318–325
37. Martins LC, Conceição FL, Muxfeldt ES et al (2012) Prevalence and associated factors of subclinical hypercortisolism in patients with resistant hypertension. J Hypertens 30:967–973
38. Václavík J, Sedlák R, Plachy M et al (2011) Addition of spironolactone in patients with resistant arterial hypertension (ASPIRANT): a randomized, double-blind, placebo-controlled trial. Hypertension 57:1069–1075
39. Zelinka T, Pacák K, Widimský J Jr (2006) Characteristics of blood pressure in pheochromocytoma. Ann N Y Acad Sci 1073:86–93

40. Muxfeldt ES, Fiszman R, de Souza F et al (2012) Appropriate time interval to repeat ambulatory blood pressure monitoring in patients with white-coat resistant hypertension. Hypertension 59:384–389
41. Krum H, Schlaich M, Whitbourn R et al (2009) Catheter-based renal sympathetic denervation for resistant hypertension: a multicentre safety and proof-of-principle cohort study. Lancet 373:1275–1281
42. Simplicity Trial Investigators (2011) Catheter-based renal sympathetic denervation for resistant hypertension: durability of blood pressure reduction out to 24 months. Hypertension 57:911–917
43. Esler MD, Krum H, Sobotka PA et al (2010) Renal sympathetic denervation in patients with treatment-resistant hypertension (the Symplicity HTN-2 trial): a randomised controlled trial. Lancet 376:1903–1909
44. Doumas M, Anyfanti P, Bakris G (2012) Should ambulatory blood pressure monitoring be mandatory for future studies in resistant hypertension: a perspective. J Hypertens 30:874–876
45. Campos-Rodriguez F, Grilo-Reina A, Perez-Ronchel J et al (2006) Effect of continuous positive airway pressure on ambulatory BP in patients with sleep apnea and hypertension: a placebo-controlled trial. Chest 129:1459–1467
46. Lozano L, Tovar JL, Sampol G et al (2010) Continuous positive airway pressure treatment in sleep apnea patients with resistant hypertension: a randomized, controlled trial. J Hypertens 28:2161–2168
47. Marui FR, Bombig MT, Francisco YA et al (2010) Assessment of resistant hypertension with home blood pressure monitoring. Arq Bras Cardiol 95:536–540
48. Nasothimiou EG, Tzamouranis D, Roussias LG et al (2011) Home versus ambulatory blood pressure monitoring in the diagnosis of clinic resistant and true resistant hypertension. J Hum Hypertens Nov 11 Epub ahead of print

Factors Predicting Blood Pressure Response to Treatment

9

Csaba Farsang

In general, the **effects of drugs** are basically determined by pharmacokinetic and pharmacodynamic properties of the drug and by special characteristics of the patient who would be treated.

9.1 Drug-Related Factors

Although they have important effects on drug actions, the manufacturing process-related characteristics (different formulations—injections, solutions, tablets, capsules—retardation methods) will not be discussed here.

The effects of drugs are mainly characterized by their pharmacokinetic and pharmacodynamics properties. As a simplification, pharmacokinetic properties of drugs describe what the organism does to the drug, and pharmacodynamics characteristics show what the drug does to the patient.

Pharmacokinetics. This depends on the way of administration (intravenously, intramuscularly, orally), absorption, distribution in different compartments of the body, metabolism-, and excretion-related processes. Apart from emergency situations when medications should be given intravenously [1], antihypertensive therapy means oral administration of drugs. Sublingual administration of the short-acting nifedipine in high dose (20–80 mg) was related to serious side effects; therefore, it is no longer advised for patients with hypertensive urgency [2].

Pharmacodynamics. In general, a drug acts when it reaches its target: receptors, enzymes, membrane ion channels, aquaporins, transport proteins, and antigens. The *effect* depends on the dose/concentration of the drug as described by the equation: $E = f(t, D)$, where t stands for the time elapsed from administration and

C. Farsang (✉)
St. Imre Teaching Hospital, Budapest, Tétényi u 12-16, H-1115, Hungary
e-mail: hunghyp@t-online.hu

G. Mancia (ed.), *Resistant Hypertension*, DOI: 10.1007/978-88-470-5415-8_9,

D for the dose. Consequently, the effect increases, reaches the peak, and then decreases. This process can be described in pharmacological/clinicopharmacological studies by the following characteristics: time-to-peak effect, (t_p), maximum concentration/effect ($C_{\max}$), elimination half-life ($t_{½}$), and area under concentration–time curve (AUC). *Efficacy* ($E_{\max}$) refers to the maximum response achievable from a drug, for example, it is the ability of a drug to reproduce a desired effect in expert hands and under ideal circumstances. *Potency* is a measure of drug activity expressed in terms of the amount required to produce an effect of given intensity. *Effectiveness* relates to the ability of a drug to produce a beneficial effect obtained under typical use circumstances when adherence is usually not 100 % [3–6]. *Efficiency* is the extent to which time or therapeutic effort is well used for the intended task (e.g., normalization of blood pressure).

Antihypertensive drugs acting on cell membrane receptors. These **receptors** are definitive structures developed in cell/intracellular membranes. They have the ability to bind endogenous ligands [e.g., acetylcholine, epinephrine, norepinephrine, dopamine, angiotensin II, vasopressin, endothelins, serotonin (5-OH-tryptamine), etc.,] or exogenously administered drugs. Several receptors are target of antihypertensive drugs. The alpha-1 and alpha-2 adrenoceptors, the beta-1 and beta-2 adrenergic receptors, the imidazoline I1 receptor, the angiotensin II AT1 receptor, the prorenin–renin receptors, and less frequently the $5HT_{1A}$ receptors are target of antihypertensive drugs which inhibit or stimulate these receptors. Apart from dose-related properties, the agonist effects of these drugs are related to the characteristics of their binding (specificity, strength, duration, reversibility) to these receptors and the density/number of these receptors in the cell membranes of the target organs.

Antihypertensive drugs acting on intracellular steroid receptors. Aldosterone antagonists (spironolactone, eplerenone) decrease BP by binding to intracellular mineralocorticoid receptors and inhibit the expression of receptor-related Na^+/K^+-ATPase enzyme and thereby the reabsorption of Na^+ and retention of K^+ in the renal distal tubuli. Consequently, the Na^+ and Ca^{++} contents of vascular smooth muscles decrease that induces vasodilation and decrease total peripheral resistance and BP.

Antihypertensive drugs acting on enzymes. The most important examples of these drugs are the angiotensin-converting **enzyme** inhibitors (ACEI). In monotherapy or in most of the patients, in combination with diuretics or calcium antagonists (CCB), they are frequently used in everyday practice.

Drugs acting on ion channels. There are two, ligand-dependent, and voltage-dependent types of *calcium channels*. The voltage-dependent **ion channels** have different subtypes: L, P/Q, N, R, and T. The calcium channel blockers (CCB), usually called as calcium antagonists, are frequently used for antihypertensive therapy. They are mostly inhibiting the L-type calcium channels and have three main chemical structures: dihydropyridines, phenylalkylamines, and benzothiazepines. These calcium channels are distributed throughout in the body and have specific structures characterized by different subunits (alpha, beta, delta). The CCBs bind to these subunits, mostly to the alpha-1, and inhibit the release of Ca^{++}

from intracellular stores and the entry of Ca^{++} from extracellular to intracellular space, resulting relaxation of vascular smooth muscles and decreasing total peripheral resistance and thereby blood pressure. The *potassium channels* also have different types: voltage-dependent, Ca^{++}-activated, ATP-sensitive, and ACh-sensitive ones and inward rectifiers. For antihypertensive therapy, the potassium channel openers (e.g., diazoxide, minoxidil) are in clinical practice; these are frequently referred to as "direct vasodilators."

Drugs acting on transport proteins. For the antihypertensive therapy, the $Na^{+}K^{+}2Cl^{-}$ cotransporter in the ascending limb of Henle's loop of renal tubuli for loop diuretics (e.g., furosemide) only in patients with advanced renal disease, and the $Na^{+}Cl^{-}$ transporter in the early distal tubuli, as target of thiazide-type diuretics (DIU) should be mentioned.

Drug interactions. Drugs may influence the effect of each other by several **synergistic mechanisms**: They could have an effect on the same or closely coupled macromolecule (e.g., on receptors or receptor mosaics), on the same cells, on the same or different signal transduction, and on different cells. The result can be an **antagonism** (competitive or non-competitive) or a **stimulation** (additive or potentiation synergism) of the antihypertensive action. An example for the additive synergism/potentiation is the combination of an ACEI/ARB with a DIU or with a CCB, or a DIU with a BBL [7].

9.2 Patient-Related Factors

There are several characteristics of patients that may influence the antihypertensive effects of drugs. Patients' age, gender, height and body weight, and also body composition might influence their responses to a drug that is commonly accepted. However, this may not be relevant to hypertensives with coronary heart disease as in the INVEST Study 12-month BP control was not affected by gender, prior smoking, age, dyslipidemia, or obesity [8]. *Smoking*, by activating the release of enzymes, accelerates drug metabolism. Stress, circadian, and ultradian physiologic rhythms closely connected to release of hormones and neurotransmitters such as catecholamines and cortisol also change responses to drugs because of inhibiting or accelerating drug metabolism. *Alcohol*, by interacting with several drugs, including antihypertensives, may change the patient's responses to medication. From among patient-related factors, only the most important or frequent ones are shortly described below.

Psychological factors, for example, aversion to drugs, previous experience with medicines, forgetfulness, level of education, expectations regarding the outcome of the therapy, the family's influence on patients' actions, and the communication with healthcare providers, are those having important influence on response to therapy. *Living conditions* (employment, housing, urban or rural environment) frequently modify patients' attitude to comply with instructions of the treating physicians. One of the most important factors in this respect is the *patients'*

***adherence* to therapy**, which is affected by several factors, for example, smoking, depression, feeling sad or blue for 2 weeks or more, and eating fast food ≥2 times per week, number of drugs to be taken together, frequency of drug administration (once or more times a day), side effects, price of drugs, even the color of the pills, frequency of medical visits, doctors' and nurses' attention, concomitant diseases, and seriousness of the disease. It has also been proved that **fixed** (or single pill) **combinations** are more effective than high-dose monotherapies, or two- or three-drug regimens [9–12]. It is known that in patients with good adherence, the blood pressure (BP) response to antihypertensive drugs was better, and consequently, they had less and milder cardiovascular (CV), cerebrovascular (CVA) or renal events or organ damage (left ventricular hypertrophy, angina pectoris, acute coronary syndrome, transient ischemic attack, stroke, microalbuminuria, proteinuria, end-stage renal disease), and less mortality rate than in those whose adherence was worse [13].

Lifestyle properties and *dietary habits* may also influence drug responses. In patients with frequent stress situations, the antihypertensive effects of drugs inhibiting sympathetic efferentation (e.g., beta-blockers) are enhanced [14].

False tolerance due to salt and water retention can inhibit hypotensive effect of sympatholytic drugs when they are given in long-term monotherapy which can be overcome by diuretics (DIU) [15]. Also, patients who consume high amount of salt respond better to diuretics than those with low-salt diet [16, 17].

Timing of drug administration can also be important as bedtime taking was advantageous for reducing CV risk in patients with chronic kidney diseases [18]. Evening administration of drugs can also change the non-dipping pattern to dipping and thereby improve BP control [19].

Blood pressure level and hypertension-induced *target organ damage* are also important determinants of blood pressure response to drugs. In patients with higher BP, the same dose of drug is more effective than in those with lower BP [20].

Systemic atherosclerosis characterized by increased **pulse wave velocity** (PWV) may predict response to some antihypertensive drugs [21]. Atherosclerosis and probably **serum cholesterol** level may also have influence on antihypertensive effect of drugs. Nitrendipine, a CCB, significantly decreased systolic BP in patients with low serum cholesterol level, but not in those with high cholesterol [22]. The **state of the brain**, described by structural and functional brain indices (combined ratings of ventricle and sulcal size and white matter hyperintensities) of MRI and PET, may also be a predictor of blood pressure response to atenolol or lisinopril [23].

Neurohumoral status of patients has also influence on the effect of different types of antihypertensive treatment [24]. The activation of the **renin–angiotensin system** (RAS) may predict the blood pressure response as the effect of drugs inhibiting RAS (ACEI, ARB, and BBL) was larger and that of DIU was smaller than in those patients with normal or low PRA [25, 26]. However, in a study, pretreatment plasma renin activity (PRA) and plasma norepinephrine did not predict the antihypertensive effect of captopril or diltiazem [27].

In those patients with increased production of aldosterone (e.g., patients with Conn's syndrome or other forms of hypermineralocorticism), the antihypertensive effect of aldosterone antagonists (spironolactone, eplerenone) is enhanced. Similarly, in those patients with high sympathetic activity, the antihypertensive effect of drugs centrally inhibiting **sympathetic efferentation** (alpha-2 adrenoceptor agonists, imidazoline I1 receptor agonists) or blocking the effects of the peripherally released neurotransmitter norepinephrine (BBL, alpha-1 blockers) is more pronounced than of those having no direct action on this system. Average *daytime heart rate*, as a sign of enhanced sympathetic activity, determined by 24-h ABPM, was also found to be a good predictor of BP response to BBL or ACEIs [28].

Genetic determinants of blood pressure response to antihypertensive agents have intensively been investigated. Because drug metabolism is genetically determined, race may affect responses. This is known as **genetic polymorphism**. It results in racial differences in response to some antihypertensive agents. In Afro-American people usually having a low plasma renin activity, the antihypertensive effect of CCBs or DIUs was better than the effect of agents inhibiting RAS, such as ACEI, ARB, and BBL [29]. **Pharmacogenomic research** revealed large diversities in response to drugs of patients with different gene polymorphism. Among them, acetylation polymorphism (slow or fast acetylators influencing drug elimination processes), and the genes coding for angiotensinogen, angiotensin-converting enzyme, and the angiotensin II AT1 receptor should be mentioned. Earlier it was found that in patients with I/I, polymorphism responded better to ACE inhibitors than those with D/D [30, 31]. A recent review showed that the conventional genetic variants of the system (i.e., the ACE I/D, AGT M235T, AT1 A1166C, and AT2 variant) were not associated with antihypertensive effects by RAS blockade. On the other hand, significant associations were found for AGT rs7079, AT1 haplotype, REN, and ACE2 [32]. Other genetic variants, such as the G-protein-coupled receptor kinase 4 polymorphisms, have also been shown to have important effect on blood pressure response to dietary salt reduction [33].

As a conclusion, at present, testing the activity of RAS or the genetic polymorphisms cannot be recommended in selecting the antihypertensive drug for a certain subject, but future research certainly would help identifying the most useful medication of a patient.

Concomitant diseases of patients affecting absorption (gastrointestinal diseases), metabolism (liver diseases), or excretion (liver or renal diseases) of drugs have also important effects on blood pressure responses. These will not be discussed here. The selection of the proper antihypertensive drug may be influenced by several factors including concomitant diseases [34]. Diabetes mellitus is one of the most frequent comorbidites in hypertensive patients, and in the INVEST Study, it was a good predictor of insufficient blood pressure response to antihypertensive therapy [8].

Concomitant therapies with non-cardiovascular drugs and *combinations of different types of antihypertensive drugs* may also influence pharmacokinetic/ pharmacodynamics properties of these drugs, as described elsewhere [7, 35].

References

1. Agabiti Rosei E, Salvetti M, Farsang C (2011) Treatment of hypertensive urgencies and emergencies. In: Narkiewicz K (ed) European society hypertension clinical practice newsletters update, pp 55–57
2. Grossman E, Messerli FH, Rodzicki T et al (1996) Should a moratorium be placed on sublingual nifedipine capsules given for hypertensive emergencies and pseudo-emergencies? JAMA 276:1328–1331
3. Israili ZH (1979) Correlation of pharmacological effects with plasma levels of antihypertensive drugs in man. Annu Rev Pharmacol Toxicol 19:25–52
4. Holford NHG, Sheiner LB (1981) Understanding the dose-effect relationship: clinical application of pharmacokinetic-pharmacodynamic models. Clin Pharmacokinet 6:429–453
5. Walker MG, Page CP, Hoffman BF, Curtis M (2006) Integrated pharmacology, 3rd edn. Mosby, St. Louis
6. Höcht C, Mayer MA, Opezzo AW et al (2008) Pharmacokinetic-pharmacodynamic modeling of antihypertensive drugs: its application to clinical practice. Rev Argent Cardiol 76:305–312
7. van Zwieten PA, Alföldi S, Farsang C (2011) Beneficial combinations of two or more antihypertensive agents. In: Narkiewicz K (ed) European society of hypertension clinical practice newsletters update, pp 33–34
8. Cooper-DeHoff RM, Handberg EM, Bristol HA et al (2002) Characteristics predicting blood pressure responses in 22,599 patients with hypertension and coronary artery disease: the international verapamil SR/trandolapril study. Am J Hypertens Part 2 15(4):238
9. Grégoire JP, Moisan J, Guibert R et al (2001) Tolerability of antihypertensive drugs in a community-based setting. Clin Ther 23:715–726
10. Aggarwal B, Mosca L (2010) Lifestyle and psychosocial risk factors predict non-adherence to medication. Ann Behav Med 40:228–233
11. Elijovich F, Laffer C (2009) A role for single-pill triple therapy in hypertension. Ther Adv Cardiovasc Dis 3:231–240
12. Wald DS, Law M, Morris JK et al (2009) Combination therapy versus monotherapy in reducing blood pressure: meta-analysis on 11,000 participants from 42 trials. Am J Med 122:290–300
13. Mancia G, Grassi G (2010) Management of essential hypertension. Br Med Bull 94:189–199
14. Lopez-Sendon J, Swedberg K, McMurray J et al (2004) Expert consensus document on β-adrenergic receptor blockers. The task force on beta-blockers of the European society of cardiology. Eur Heart J 25:1341–1362
15. Dustan HP (1983) Causes of inadequate response to antihypertensive drugs. Volume factors. Hypertension 5:I26–I30
16. Buter H, Hemmelder MH, Navis G et al (1998) The blunting of the antiproteinuric efficacy of ACE inhibition by high sodium intake can be restored by hydrochlorothiazide. Nephrol Dial Transplant 13:1682
17. Luft FC, Weinberger MH (1988) Review of salt restriction and the response to antihypertensive drugs. Satellite symposium on calcium antagonists. Hypertension 11:I229
18. Hermida RC, Ayala DE,Mojón A et al (2011) Bedtime dosing of antihypertensive medications reduces cardiovascular risk in CKD. J Am Soc Nephrol 12:2313–2321
19. Almirall J, Comas L, Martínez-Ocaña JC, Roca S, Arnau A (2012) Effects of chronotherapy on blood pressure control in non-dipper patients with refractory hypertension. Nephrol Dial Transplant 27:1855–1859
20. Sparrow D, Garvey AJ, Rosner B (1982) Factors in predicting blood pressure change. Circulation 65:789–794
21. Protogerou A, Blacher J, Stergiou GS et al (2009) Blood pressure response under chronic antihypertensive drug therapy: the role of aortic stiffness in the REASON (Preterax in regression of arterial stiffness in a controlled double-blind) study. Am Coll Cardiol 53:445–451

22. Megnien JL, Simon A, Mikaberidze E et al (2001) Do arterial effects of antihypertensive drugs depend on subject's serum cholesterol? J Cardiovasc Pharmacol 38:520–528
23. Richard J, Jennings JR, Muldoon MF et al (2008) Brain imaging findings predict blood pressure response to pharmacological treatment. Hypertension 52:1113–1119
24. Evans RR, Davis WR, Wallace JM et al (1990) Humoral factors determining the blood pressure response to converting enzyme inhibition and calcium channel blockade. Am J Hypertens 3(8 Pt 1):605–610
25. Turner ST, Schwartz GL, Chapman AB et al (2010) Plasma renin activity predicts blood pressure responses to β- blocker and thiazide diuretic as monotherapy and add-on therapy for hypertension. Am J Hypertens 23:1014–1022
26. Canzanello VJ, Baranco-Pryor E, Rahbari-Oskoui F et al (2008) Predictors of blood pressure response to the angiotensin receptor blocker candesartan in essential hypertension. Am J Hypertens 21:61–66
27. Robert R, Evans R, Davis WR et al (1990) Humoral factors determining the blood pressure response to converting enzyme inhibition and calcium channel blockade. Am J Hypertens 3(28):605–610
28. Owens PE, Lyons S, O'Brien E (1998) Can heart rate predict blood pressure response to antihypertensive drug therapy? J Hum Hypertens 12:229–233
29. Flack JM, Nasser SA, Levy PD (2011) Therapy of hypertension in African Americans disclosures. Am J Cardiovasc Drugs 11:83–92
30. Stephen T, Turner L, Schwartz GL et al (2001) Antihypertensive pharmacogenetics: getting the right drug into the right patient. J Hypertens 19:1–11
31. Materson BJ (2007) Variability in response to antihypertensive drugs. Am J Med 120 (4 Suppl 1):S10–S20
32. Konoshita Y (2011) The genomic disease outcome consortium (G-DOC) study investigators. Do genetic variants of the renin-angiotensin system predict blood pressure response to renin-angiotensin system–blocking drugs? A systematic review of pharmacogenomics in the renin-angiotensin system. Curr Hypertens Rep 13:356–361
33. Rayner B, Ramesar R, Steyn K et al (2012) G-protein-coupled receptor kinase 4 polymorphisms predict blood pressure response to dietary modification in Black patients with mild-to-moderate hypertension. J Hum Hypertens 26:334–339
34. Mancia G, Laurent S, Agabiti-Rosei E et al (2009) Reappraisal of European guidelines on hypertension management: a European society of hypertension (ESH) task force document. J Hypertens 27:2121–2158
35. van Zwieten PA, Alföldi S, Farsang C (2011) Interactions between antihypertensive agents and other drugs. In: Narkiewicz K (ed) European society of hypertension clinical practice newsletters update, pp 31–32

Treatment of Resistant Hypertension. Which Additional Antihypertensive Drugs?

10

Michel Burnier, Antoinette Pechère Bertschi and Gregoire Wuerzner

10.1 Introduction

According to the latest European and American guidelines, hypertension should be considered as resistant if "BP remains $\geq$140/90 mmHg despite treatment with at least three drugs (including a diuretic) in adequate doses and after exclusion of spurious hypertension such as isolated office hypertension and failure to use large cuffs on large arms" [1, 2]. Among the many causes of resistant hypertension discussed in a previous chapter, several are linked directly to the quality of the drug therapy. As shown in Table 10.1, various aspects of the medical treatment should be considered when evaluating a new patient with resistant hypertension. Is the patient receiving the appropriate drug doses? Are drug combinations adequate and effective? Is the patient adherent to therapy and finally what other medical or non-pharmacological therapies could be proposed to improve the control of blood pressure? The purpose of this chapter is to discuss these various aspects which, in our opinion, are crucial to consider and correct before starting costly investigations searching for secondary causes of hypertension or even envisaging renal denervation.

M. Burnier (✉) · G. Wuerzner
Service of Nephrology and Hypertension, University Hospital,
Rued du Bugnon 17, 1011 Lausanne, Switzerland
e-mail: michel.burnier@chuv.ch

A. P. Bertschi
Unit of Hypertension, Departments of Specialties of Medicine and Community Medicine and Primary Care and Emergency Medicine, University Hospital, Geneva, Switzerland

G. Mancia (ed.), *Resistant Hypertension*, DOI: 10.1007/978-88-470-5415-8_10,

Table 10.1 Medical therapy–related causes of resistant hypertension

Inadequate dosages
Inappropriate drug combinations
Inappropriate diuretic therapy or dosage
Medication intolerance
Drug interactions (for example, non-steroidal anti-inflammatory drugs, sympathomimetics, contraceptives, ciclosporine, corticosteroids…)
Drug adherence

10.2 Suboptimal Medical Regimens: A Common Error

10.2.1 Drug Doses

Although the dose–response curve of antihypertensive drugs is generally considered to be relatively flat, there is a clear and significant difference in the fall in blood pressure induced by half doses of the five categories of blood pressure–lowering drugs commonly used for hypertension management when compared with either a regular or a double dose of the same compound [3]. Thus, according to a review of clinical studies, differences of up to 10 mmHg systolic blood pressure can be obtained depending on the dose of the prescribed agent [3]. In a review of cases of resistant hypertension referred to a tertiary care center, a suboptimal medical regimen was the most frequent cause of apparent resistance to treatment, representing about 40 % of the clinical situations. In most cases, an optimization of the treatment, in general adaptation of the diuretics, resulted in a significant improvement in blood pressure control [4, 5]. The reluctance to increase the drug doses when blood pressure is not controlled is perhaps due to the dose–response relationship of the occurrence of side effects which is clearly steeper in particular with diuretics, calcium channel blockers, and beta-blockers [3]. In contrast, increasing the dose of a blocker of the renin–angiotensin system (RAS) is associated with little if any increase in the prevalence of side effects [3]. There is therefore no need to underdose these agents as a more complete blockade of the system may lead to greater clinical benefits in terms of blood pressure and target organ damage.

10.2.2 Drug Duration of Action

Another common issue in the medical therapy of resistant hypertension is the duration of action of drugs. Most new antihypertensive drugs have been developed as once-a-day drug. However, if drugs are marketed for a once-daily administration, not all of them are truly covering the 24 h of the day [6]. Administration of a short-acting antihypertensive agent may lead to suboptimal control of blood pressure during certain periods of the day, mainly in the evening and early morning, and hence apparent resistance to therapy. Thus, it may be important to consider the trough-to-peak ratio of the prescribed drugs in patients with uncontrolled hypertension, and a better coverage of the 24 h may often need the prescription of an evening dose. In the context of resistant hypertension, physicians should rather prescribe drugs with a very long duration of action which are truly once-a-day agent. This will not only improve blood pressure control but also simplify the treatment regimen and might provide additional benefits to lower the cardiovascular risk as suggested in a recent analysis [7].

10.2.3 Drug Combinations

Blood pressure control of patients with resistant hypertension can also be improved by adapting the combination of antihypertensive drugs. As mentioned in guidelines, the major classes of blood pressure–lowering drugs can be combined with each other in order to increase their efficacy [1, 2]. Indeed, due to the complexity of the mechanisms leading to hypertension, combining drugs with different pathophysiological targets increases the percentage of patients adequately controlled. In a recent meta-analysis of 42 trials involving more than 10,000 hypertensive patients, Wald et al. [8] have found that combining two antihypertensive drugs at low dose produced an extra blood pressure reduction five times greater than doubling the dose of one of the drug. Thus, physicians should be cautious not to prescribe two drugs from the same class of agents or two agents with the same mechanism of action (for example, two blockers of the renin–angiotensin system). Some would argue that combining an angiotensin-converting enzyme (ACE) inhibitor and an angiotensin II receptor blocker (ARB) or a renin inhibitor may lead to a more complete blockade of the system and to slightly greater decrease in blood pressure in hypertension [9–11]. Though some minor additional benefits on blood pressure have been reported with such combinations [11], the long-term use of these associations did not show any clear clinical benefits and might rather increase the risk of cardiovascular and renal complication as demonstrated in the ONTARGET and ALTITUDE trials [12, 13]. Moreover, using RAS blockers at their optimal dose may actually produce the same effect on blood pressure than combining two RAS blockers [14]. At last, in patients in whom hypertension was not controlled by full-dose ARB monotherapy, Stergiou et al. [15] have shown that addition of a diuretic or a calcium antagonist provided significant additional antihypertensive effects and the antihypertensive effects of the ARB–diuretic and the ARB–calcium antagonist combinations were superior to that of the ARB–ACE inhibitor combination further emphasizing the recommendation to favor the prescription of antihypertensive agents with different mechanisms of action.

Recent large clinical trials have now demonstrated that all drug combinations are not equally effective in terms of organ protection and prevention of cardiovascular and renal complications although their impact on systemic blood pressure is almost comparable. Thus, the results of the Anglo-Scandinavian Cardiac Outcomes Trial (ASCOT) have demonstrated the superiority of combining an ACE inhibitor and a calcium antagonist in comparison with a beta-blocker–diuretic combination [16]. More recently, the association of an ACE inhibitor and a calcium antagonist was also found to be superior to the ACE inhibitor–diuretic combination at least in patients at high cardiovascular risk [17]. Of note, in the ASCOT trial, being randomized to perindopril ± amlodipine significantly reduced the risk of resistant hypertension [relative risk: 0.57 (0.50–0.60)] [18]. Thus, today, two drug associations are widely used for the management of hypertension, that is, RAS blockers combined with a diuretic and RAS blockers associated with a calcium antagonist. Together with their antihypertensive efficacy, these drug combinations are very useful in the context of resistant hypertension as they also offer the possibility to simplify the treatment regimen and to reduce the pill burden, hence increasing drug adherence.

10.2.4 Drug Interactions

Drug interactions are also important to consider in the medical management of resistant hypertension. Several drugs have the potential to increase blood pressure either directly or by blunting the efficacy of antihypertensive agents. This is the case, for example, of non-steroidal anti-inflammatory drugs (NSAIDs) which cause sodium retention, enhance the vasoconstrictor response to vasopressor hormones and antagonize the effects of other antihypertensive drugs essentially diuretics and RAS blockers [19–21]. Interestingly, NSAIDs do not affect the blood pressure response to calcium antagonists which therefore are the drugs of choice if pain therapy is absolutely necessary [20]. The use of oral contraceptives has also been associated with an increased risk of uncontrolled hypertension in hypertensive women, and blood pressure control can be improved by adapting the contraception strategy [22]. Other common drugs involved in the development of resistant hypertension are sympathomimetic amines such as nasal spray and oral decongestants that contain alpha-adrenergic vasoactive compounds. Corticosteroids, cyclosporine, and recombinant erythropoietin are also frequently prescribed drug-causing resistant hypertension.

10.3 Diuretics in Resistant Hypertension: A Critical Issue

In patients with resistant hypertension, volume overload due to salt and water retention belongs to the most common physiological mechanisms leading to the rise in blood pressure despite medical therapy. An excessive dietary salt intake not only raises blood pressure by increasing intravascular volume but also reduces the efficacy of antihypertensive drugs mainly diuretics and blockers of the renin–angiotensin system. Conversely, all antihypertensive agents are more effective when patients follow a sodium restricted diet [23]. In this respect, Pimenta et al. have shown that reducing salt intake from 250 to 50 mmol/day resulted in a marked and significant BP in subjects with resistant hypertension [24]. On ambulatory blood pressure monitoring, the fall in BP achieved 22/9 mmHg, respectively, for systolic and diastolic BPs. Although these results were gathered on a very small number of subjects ($n = 12$), they further emphasize the importance of salt intake in the management of resistant hypertension.

Many patients referred for resistant hypertension do not receive an appropriate diuretic or diuretic dose. Thus, in patients with a normal glomerular filtration rate (GFR), prescription of a loop diuretic may be inadequate as the acute natriuretic effect is followed by a long-standing antinatriuresis. Hence, it is difficult to induce a negative sodium balance with these agents. Loop diuretics should be considered only for patients with reduced renal function, usually an estimated GFR below 30 ml/min. More recently, there has been intense discussion on whether thiazide diuretics are really the most appropriate and effective diuretics and whether physicians should prefer chlorthalidone or eventually indapamide rather than hydrochlorothiazide (HCTZ) for the management of hypertensive patients. Two meta-analyses were recently conducted which compared the antihypertensive efficacy as well as the impact on the prevention of cardiovascular events of HCTZ and chlorthalidone [25, 26]. The latter was found to be more potent than HCTZ at least when used at standard dose ranges [25]. This analysis therefore confirms the results of a randomized, single-blinded, 8-week active treatment, crossover study comparing chlorthalidone 12.5 mg/day (force-titrated to 25 mg/day) and hydrochlorothiazide 25 mg/day (force-titrated to 50 mg/day) in untreated hypertensive patients [27]. In this study, chlorthalidone was superior to HCTZ when blood pressure was measured using ambulatory blood pressure monitoring. In the second meta-analysis, chlorthalidone was found to be superior to HCTZ in preventing cardiovascular events [26]. These results are now further confirmed by the demonstration that combining an ARB with chlorthalidone produces a greater decrease in blood pressure than the same ARB combined with HCTZ [28].

The administration of a diuretic acting at a specific site along the renal tubules has been shown to be associated with counter-regulatory mechanisms leading to an upregulation of sodium transporters both in upstream and in downstream segments of the nephron [29, 30]. This leads to a compensatory increase in renal sodium reabsorption which limits the natriuretic response to the administered diuretic. For this reason, it has been suggested to combine diuretics acting at different sites in order to increase the efficacy of the therapeutic strategy [31]. The strategy of sequential nephron blockade has recently been investigated in patients with resistant hypertension referred to a tertiary center and compared to a sequential blockade of the renin–angiotensin system [32]. In this study, 167 patients with an elevated ambulatory blood pressure (mean 150/93 mmHg) despite a triple therapy of irbesartan 300 mg, amlodipine 5 mg, and HCTZ 12.5 mg were randomized to sequential nephron blockade which consisted of the step-by-step addition of spironolactone 25 mg followed by furosemide 20–40 mg and amiloride 5 mg or sequential blockade of the renin–angiotensin system with the sequential addition

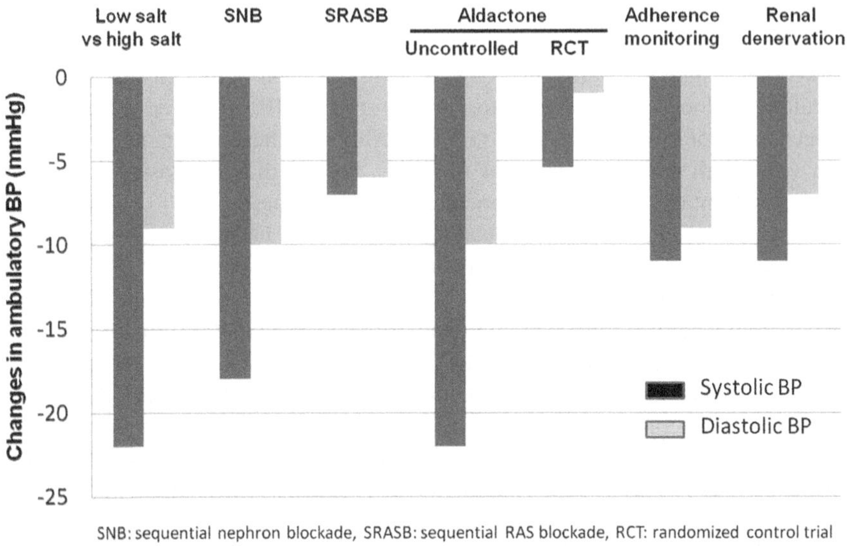

Fig. 10.1 Comparative effects on ambulatory systolic and diastolic blood pressures of various therapeutic approaches in patients with resistant hypertension. (Data from [24, 32, 39, 48, 53, 57])

of ramipril 5–10 mg and bisoprolol 5 mg. After 12 weeks of therapy, the mean ambulatory BP decrease was, respectively, 18 and 10 mmHg for systolic and diastolic BPs with sequential nephron blockade versus 7 and 6 mmHg with sequential blockade of the RAS (Fig. 10.1). These results suggest that combining diuretics at low doses may be interesting to increase the percentage of patients with resistant hypertension reaching the BP target as 58 % of the patients receiving the sequential nephron blockade reached the ambulatory BP target of <135/85 mmHg. Importantly, the incidence of side effects was low, and very few patients discontinued therapy. Taken together, these data suggest that sequential nephron blockade may be an interesting approach in patients with resistant hypertension.

10.4 What is the Role of Mineralocorticoid Receptor Blockade?

The exact mechanisms whereby blood pressure is more difficult to control in some patients but not in others are not completely understood. Several large epidemiological studies or post hoc analysis of large trials have investigated the determinants of resistant hypertension, and some factors such as diabetes, left ventricular hypertrophy, male sex, and raised body mass index, fasting glucose, and alcohol intake have been regularly identified [18, 33–35]. Some of these parameters such as metabolic syndrome are associated with higher levels of plasma aldosterone [36], and in the assessment of 279 consecutive patients with resistant hypertension, Gaddam et al. have reported significantly higher plasma aldosterone levels among patients with resistant hypertension, suggesting that plasma aldosterone levels may play a role in the blood pressure resistance even in patients with sleep apnea syndrome [35, 37].

For these many reasons, several investigators have investigated the role of mineralocorticoid receptor blockade with Aldactone on blood pressure control in subjects with resistant hypertension. Several studies actually reported significant falls in blood pressure upon administration of Aldactone in resistant hypertension. The largest experience has probably been acquired in the ASCOT blood pressure arm where Aldactone has been used as 4th line of treatment in patients not responding to a triple therapy [38]. In this trial, more than one-third of patients had the criteria of resistant hypertension and 1,411 received 25 mg of Aldactone on top of their treatment. With the addition of Aldactone, a significant fall in blood pressure of 22 mmHg systolic and 10 mmHg diastolic was observed (Fig. 10.1) [39]. This was confirming the data of many smaller studies [40–47]. Recently, one randomized prospective double-blind placebo-controlled study was conducted in resistant hypertension to assess the clinical impact of mineralocorticoid receptor blockade (the ASPIRANT study) [48]. In this study, 117 patients with resistant hypertension were randomized to receive either Aldactone 25 mg or a placebo on top of their triple therapy mostly RAS blockers, diuretics, and calcium antagonists. In this study, the 8-week reduction in blood pressure was 5.4 mmHg for systolic and only 1 mmHg for diastolic suggesting only a minor favorable impact on blood pressure of Aldactone (Fig. 10.1). These results contrast with those of non-randomized uncontrolled studies discussed above. Despite these conflicting data on the impact of mineralocorticoid receptor blockade in resistant hypertension, some national guidelines recommend to consider renal denervation for resistant hypertension only after having performed a therapeutic challenge with spironolactone [49].

10.5 Drug Adherence: The Crucial Step in Resistant Hypertension

Whatever the drug prescribed for the management of resistant hypertension, a major criterion of success is the ability of the patient to follow the recommendations on a daily basis (adherence) and to stay on therapy (persistence). It is well recognized that long-term drug persistence is rather low in patients treated for silent diseases such as hypertension. Thus, in a large review of phase IV studies in which drug adherence was measured by electronic monitoring, persistence was only 50 % at one year [50]. Drug adherence and persistence are essential in patients with resistant hypertension, and poor adherence to therapy is a well-recognized determinant of resistant hypertension. However, the issue is difficult to address for many reasons. Firstly, reliable and cheap diagnostic tools available to diagnose non-adherence are still lacking. Many investigators use questionnaires (such as the Morisky) or the pill count to evaluate drug adherence, but these approaches are unprecise and overestimate drug adherence [51, 52]. In hypertension, major differences of up to 25 % in drug adherence have been observed between questionnaires and the actual taking adherence measured by electronic monitoring [52]. Secondly, the percentage of drug adherence necessary to achieve in order to get a good blood pressure control in resistant hypertension has not been determined. The literature frequently analyzes data with an arbitrary cutoff of 80 %, but this figure has never been validated. At last, very few interventional studies have actually investigated prospectively the impact of drug adherence monitoring on blood pressure control.

We have used the Medication Event Monitoring System (MEMS) to measure drug adherence in patients with resistant hypertension [53]. To assess the impact of drug adherence monitoring, the triple drug therapy was remained unchanged but monitored electronically for two months. In this group of 41 patients with resistant hypertension, a low drug adherence correlated with a high diastolic blood pressure. Monitoring of drug adherence per se resulted in a significant decrease in blood pressure, respectively, by 11 mmHg systolic and 9 mmHg diastolic (Fig. 10.1). More importantly, the determination of drug adherence enabled to distinguish patients who actually needed investigations or drug adaptations because their adherence was perfect from those who rather needed an intervention on drug adherence to improve their acceptation of the treatment.

These data therefore confirm that drug adherence monitoring plays an important role in the management of resistant as it help to take more rational therapeutic decisions.

10.6 Future Drug Therapies in Resistant Hypertension

In recent years, studies have been conducted in patients with resistant hypertension investigating new medical approaches. As there is an important medical need for these high cardiovascular risk patients, endothelin receptor antagonists have been considered an interesting new therapeutic approach in this indication [54–56]. Indeed, because these patients have a high incidence of cardiovascular complications, the tolerability profile of endothelin antagonists remains favorable when compared with the global risk of target organ damages.

The DORADO study demonstrated that the addition of darusentan to a triple therapy was superior to the addition of a placebo [54]. This study included patients with an impaired renal function and proteinuria, and the addition of darusentan was also associated with a reduction in urinary protein excretion. Unfortunately, the early favorable results of darusentan in resistant hypertension were not confirmed in the latest DORADO-AC study. In this randomized controlled trial, a major placebo effect was observed at week 14, whereas at week 8, there was a significant difference between the blood pressure–lowering effect of darusentan and placebo or the alpha-blocker, guanfacine. These disturbing results were probably due to technical problems linked to the measurement of office blood pressure.

Indeed, when blood pressure was assessed using ambulatory monitoring, which avoids the placebo effect, a marked and significant effect of darusentan was observed [55]. Thus, it seems that ETA receptor blockade can provide clinical benefits in patients with resistant hypertension, but these data should be confirmed with additional well-conducted randomized trials. In terms of tolerability profile, the major side effect of darusentan was again fluid retention with a decrease in hematocrit due to hemodilution [56].

10.7 Conclusions

The investigation of patients with resistant hypertension should always start with a careful assessment of the prescribed drug therapy in order to correct the most frequent errors such as inadequate dosing, inappropriate drug combinations, and insufficient diuretic therapy. Moreover, whenever possible, drug adherence should be monitored carefully. Such an office-based non-invasive evaluation should be very cost-effective and may contribute to limit the need for costly investigations looking for secondary hypertension or renal denervation.

References

1. Mancia G, De Backer G, Dominiczak A, Cifkova R, Fagard R, Germano G, Grassi G, Heagerty AM, Kjeldsen SE, Laurent S, Narkiewicz K, Ruilope L, Rynkiewicz A, Schmieder RE, Boudier HA, Zanchetti A (2007) ESH-ESC task force on the management of arterial hypertension. 2007 ESH-ESC practice guidelines for the management of arterial hypertension: ESH-ESC task force on the management of arterial hypertension. J Hypertens 25(9):1751–1762
2. Chobanian AV, Bakris GL, Black HR, Cushman WC, Green LA, Izzo JL Jr, Jones DW, Materson BJ, Oparil S, Wright JT Jr, Roccella EJ (2003) National heart, lung, and blood institute joint national committee on prevention, detection, evaluation, and treatment of high blood pressure; national high blood pressure education program coordinating committee: the seventh report of the joint national committee on prevention, detection, evaluation and treatment of high blood pressure: the JNC 7 report. JAMA 289:2560–2571
3. Law MR, Wald NJ, Morris JK, Jordan RE (2003) Value of low dose combination treatment with blood pressure lowering drugs: analysis of 354 randomised trials. BMJ 326:1427
4. Yakovlevitch M, Black HR (1991) Resistant hypertension in a tertiary care clinic. Arch Intern Med 151:1786–1792
5. Setaro JF, Black HR (1992) Refractory hypertension. N Engl J Med 327:543–547
6. Meredith PA (1999) Trough: peak ratio and smoothness index for antihypertensive agents. Blood Press Monit 4(5):257–262
7. Burnier M, Brede Y, Lowy A (2011) Impact of prolonged antihypertensive duration of action on predicted clinical outcomes in imperfectly adherent patients: comparison of aliskiren, irbesartan and ramipril. Int J Clin Pract 65(2):127–133
8. Wald DS, Law M, Morris JK, Bestwick JP, Wald NJ (2009) Combination therapy versus monotherapy in reducing blood pressure: meta-analysis on 11,000 participants from 42 trials. Am J Med 122(3):290–300

9. Azizi M, Guyene TT, Chatellier G, Ménard J (1997) Pharmacological demonstration of the additive effects of angiotensin-converting enzyme inhibition and angiotensin II antagonism in sodium depleted healthy subjects. Clin Exp Hypertens 19(5–6):937–951
10. Azizi M, Ménard J, Bissery A, Guyenne TT, Bura-Rivière A, Vaidyanathan S, Camisasca RP (2004) Pharmacologic demonstration of the synergistic effects of a combination of the renin inhibitor aliskiren and the AT1 receptor antagonist valsartan on the angiotensin II-renin feedback interruption. J Am Soc Nephrol 15(12):3126–3133
11. Oparil S, Yarows SA, Patel S, Fang H, Zhang J, Satlin A (2007) Efficacy and safety of combined use of aliskiren and valsartan in patients with hypertension: a randomised, double-blind trial. Lancet 370:221–229 (Erratum in: Lancet 370(9598):1542, (2007))
12. ONTARGET Investigators, Yusuf S, Teo KK, Pogue J, Dyal L, Copland I, Schumacher H, Dagenais G, Sleight P, Telmisartan AC (2008) Ramipril, or both in patients at high risk for vascular events. N Engl J Med 358(15):1547–1559
13. McMurray JJ, Abraham WT, Dickstein K, Køber L, Massie BM, Aliskiren KH (2012) ALTITUDE, and the implications for ATMOSPHERE. Eur J Heart Fail 14(4):341–343
14. Meier P, Maillard MP, Meier JR, Tremblay S, Gauthier T, Burnier M (2011) Combining blockers of the renin-angiotensin system or increasing the dose of an angiotensin II receptor antagonist in proteinuric patients: a randomized triple-crossover study. J Hypertens 29(6):1228–1235
15. Stergiou GS, Makris T, Papavasiliou M, Efstathiou S, Manolis A (2005) Comparison of antihypertensive effects of an angiotensin-converting enzyme inhibitor, a calcium antagonist and a diuretic in patients with hypertension not controlled by angiotensin receptor blocker monotherapy. J Hypertens 23(4):883–889
16. Dahlöf B, Sever PS, Poulter NR, Wedel H, Beevers DG, Caulfield M, Collins R, Kjeldsen SE, Kristinsson A, McInnes GT, Mehlsen J, Nieminen M, O'Brien E, Ostergren J (2005) ASCOT Investigators. Prevention of cardiovascular events with an antihypertensive regimen of amlodipine adding perindopril as required versus atenolol adding bendroflumethiazide as required, in the Anglo-Scandinavian cardiac outcomes trial-blood pressure lowering arm (ASCOT-BPLA): a multicentre randomised controlled trial. Lancet 366(9489):895–906
17. Jamerson K, Weber MA, Bakris GL, Dahlöf B, Pitt B, Shi V, Hester A, Gupte J, Gatlin M, Velazquez EJ (2008) ACCOMPLISH trial investigators benazepril plus amlodipine or hydrochlorothiazide for hypertension in high-risk patients. N Engl J Med 359(23):2417–2428
18. Gupta AK, Nasothimiou EG, Chang CL, Sever PS, Dahlöf B, Poulter NR (2011) ASCOT investigators. Baseline predictors of resistant hypertension in the Anglo-Scandinavian cardiac outcome trial (ASCOT): a risk score to identify those at high-risk. J Hypertens 29(10):2004–2013
19. Rossat J, Maillard M, Nussberger J, Brunner HR, Burnier M (1999) Renal effects of selective cyclooxygenase-2 inhibition in normotensive salt-depleted subjects. Clin Pharmacol Ther 66(1):76–84
20. Morgan T, Anderson A (2003) The effect of nonsteroidal anti-inflammatory drugs on blood pressure in patients treated with different antihypertensive drugs. J Clin Hypertens 5(1):53–57
21. Fricker AF, Nussberger J, Meilenbrock S, Brunner HR, Burnier M (1998) Effect of indomethacin on the renal response to angiotensin II receptor blockade in healthy subjects. Kidney Int 54(6):2089–2097
22. Lubianca JN, Faccin CS, Fuchs FD (2003) Oral contraceptives: a risk factor for uncontrolled blood pressure among hypertensive women. Contraception 67(1):19–24
23. Weir MR, Chrysant SG, McCarron DA, Canossa-Terris M, Cohen JD, Gunter PA, Lewin AJ, Mennella RF, Kirkegaard LW, Hamilton JH, Weinberger MH, Weder AB (1998) Influence of race and dietary salt on the antihypertensive efficacy of an angiotensin-converting enzyme inhibitor or a calcium channel antagonist in salt-sensitive hypertensives. Hypertension 31(5):1088–1096

24. Pimenta E, Gaddam KK, Oparil S, Aban I, Husain S, Dell'Italia LJ, Calhoun DA (2009) Effects of dietary sodium reduction on blood pressure in subjects with resistant hypertension: results from a randomized trial. Hypertension 54(3):475–481
25. Peterzan MA, Hardy R, Chaturvedi N, Hughes AD (2012) Meta-analysis of dose-response relationships for hydrochlorothiazide, chlorthalidone, and bendroflumethiazide on blood pressure, serum potassium, and urate. Hypertension 59(6):1104–1109
26. Roush GC, Holford TR, Guddati AK (2012) Chlorthalidone compared with hydrochlorothiazide in reducing cardiovascular events: systematic review and network meta-analyses. Hypertension 59(6):1110–1117
27. Ernst ME, Carter BL, Goerdt CJ, Steffensmeier JJ, Phillips BB, Zimmerman MB, Bergus GR (2006) Comparative antihypertensive effects of hydrochlorothiazide and chlorthalidone on ambulatory and office blood pressure. Hypertension 47(3):352–358
28. Bakris GL, Sica D, White WB, Cushman WC, Weber MA, Handley A, Song E, Kupfer S (2012) Antihypertensive efficacy of hydrochlorothiazide versus chlorthalidone combined with azilsartan medoxomil. Am J Med [Epub ahead of print]
29. Na KY, Oh YK, Han JS, Lee JS, Earm JH, Knepper MA, Kim GH (2003) Upregulation of Na+ transporter abundances in response to chronic thiazide or loop diuretic treatment in rats. Am J Physiol Renal Physiol 284:F133–F143
30. Nielsen J, Kwon TH, Masilamani S, Beutler K, Hager H, Nielsen S, Knepper MA (2002) Sodium transporter abundance profiling in kidney: effect of spironolactone. Am J Physiol Renal Physiol 283:F923–F933
31. Knauf H, Mutschler E (1997) Sequential nephron blockade breaks resistance to diuretics in edematous states. J Cardiovasc Pharmacol 29:367–372
32. Bobrie G, Frank M, Azizi M, Peyrard S, Boutouyrie P, Chatellier G, Laurent S, Menard J, Plouin PF (2012) Sequential nephron blockade versus sequential renin-angiotensin system blockade in resistant hypertension: a prospective, randomized, open blinded endpoint study. J Hypertens 30(8):1656–1664
33. de la Sierra A, Segura J, Banegas JR, Gorostidi M, de la Cruz JJ, Armario P, Oliveras A, Ruilope LM (2011) Clinical features of 8,295 patients with resistant hypertension classified on the basis of ambulatory blood pressure monitoring. Hypertension 57(5):898–902
34. Martins LC, Figueiredo VN, Quinaglia T, Boer-Martins L, Yugar-Toledo JC, Martin JF, Demacq C, Pimenta E, Calhoun DA, Moreno H Jr (2011) Characteristics of resistant hypertension: ageing, body mass index, hyperaldosteronism, cardiac hypertrophy and vascular stiffness. J Hum Hypertens 25(9):532–538
35. Gaddam KK, Nishizaka MK, Pratt-Ubunama MN, Pimenta E, Aban I, Oparil S, Calhoun DA (2008) Characterization of resistant hypertension: association between resistant hypertension, aldosterone, and persistent intravascular volume expansion. Arch Intern Med 168(11): 1159–1164
36. Bochud M, Nussberger J, Bovet P, Maillard MR, Elston RC, Paccaud F, Shamlaye C, Burnier M (2006) Plasma aldosterone is independently associated with the metabolic syndrome. Hypertension 48(2):239–245
37. Pimenta E, Gaddam KK, Pratt-Ubunama MN, Nishizaka MK, Cofield SS, Oparil S, Calhoun DA (2007) Aldosterone excess and resistance to 24-h blood pressure control. J Hypertens 25(10):2131–2137
38. Dahlof B, Sever PS, Poulter NR et al (2005) Prevention of cardiovascular events with an antihypertensive regimen of amlodipine adding perindopril as required versus atenolol adding bendroflumethiazide as required, in the Anglo-Scandinavian cardiac outcomes trial-blood pressure lowering arm (ASCOT-BPLA): a multicentre randomized controlled trial. Lancet 366:895–906
39. Chapman N, Dobson J, Wilson S, Dahlöf B, Sever PS, Wedel H, Poulter NR (2007) Anglo-Scandinavian cardiac outcomes trial investigators. Effect of spironolactone on blood pressure in subjects with resistant hypertension. Hypertension 49(4):839–845

40. Engbaek M, Hjerrild M, Hallas J, Jacobsen IA (2010) The effect of low-dose spironolactone on resistant hypertension. J Am Soc Hypertens 4(6):290–294
41. Alvarez–Alvarez B, Abad-Cardiel M, Fernandez-Cruz A, Martell-Claros N (2010) Management of resistant arterial hypertension: role of spironolactone versus double blockade of the renin-angiotensin-aldosterone system. J Hypertens 28(11):2329–2335
42. Ouzan J, Perault C, Lincoff AM, Carre E, Mertes M (2002) The role of spironolactone in the treatment of patients with refractory hypertension. Am J Hypertens 15:333–339
43. Nishizaka MK, Zaman MA, Calhoun DA (2003) Efficacy of low-dose spironolactone in subjects with resistant hypertension. Am J Hypertens 16:925–930
44. Sharabi Y, Adler E, Shamis A, Nussinovitch N, Markovitz A, Grossman E (2006) Efficacy of add-on aldosterone receptor blocker in uncontrolled hypertension. Am J Hypertens 19:750–755
45. Lane DA, Shah S, Beevers DG (2007) Low-dose spironolactone in the management of resistant hypertension: a surveillance study. J Hypertens 25:891–894
46. de Souza F, Muxfeldt E, Fiszman R, Salles G (2010) Efficacy of spironolactone therapy in patients with true resistant hypertension. Hypertension 55:147–152
47. Gaddam K, Pimenta E, Thomas SJ, Cofield SS, Oparil S, Harding SM, Calhoun DA (2010) Spironolactone reduces severity of obstructive sleep apnoea in patients with resistant hypertension: a preliminary report. J Hum Hypertens 24(8):532–537
48. Václavík J, Sedlák R, Plachy M, Navrátil K, Plásek J, Jarkovsky J, Václavík T, Husár R, Kociánová E, Táborsky M (2011) Addition of spironolactone in patients with resistant arterial hypertension (ASPIRANT): a randomized, double-blind, placebo-controlled trial. Hypertension 57(6):1069–1075
49. Pathak A, Girerd X, Azizi M, Benamer H, Halimi JM, Lantelme P, Lefèvre T, Sapoval M (2012) French society of hypertension; French society of cardiology; working group on atheroma, interventional cardiology; French society of radiology. Expert consensus: renal denervation for the treatment of arterial hypertension. Arch Cardiovasc Dis 105(6–7):386–393
50. Vrijens B, Vincze G, Kristanto P, Urquhart J, Burnier M (2008) Adherence to prescribed antihypertensive drug treatments: longitudinal study of electronically compiled dosing histories. BMJ 336(7653):1114–1117
51. Shi L, Liu J, Koleva Y, Fonseca V, Kalsekar A, Pawaskar M (2010) Concordance of adherence measurement using self-reported adherence questionnaires and medication monitoring devices. Pharmacoeconomics 28(12):1097–1107
52. Hamilton GA (2003) Measuring adherence in a hypertension clinical trial. Eur J Cardiovasc Nurs 2(3):219–228
53. Burnier M, Schneider MP, Chioléro A, Stubi CL, Brunner HR (2001) Electronic compliance monitoring in resistant hypertension: the basis for rational therapeutic decisions. J Hypertens 19(2):335–341
54. Weber MA, Black H, Bakris G, Krum H, Linas S, Weiss R, Linseman JV, Wiens BL, Warren MS, Lindholm LH (2009) A selective endothelin-receptor antagonist to reduce blood pressure in patients with treatment-resistant hypertension: a randomised, double-blind, placebo-controlled trial. Lancet 374(9699):1423–1431
55. Bakris GL, Lindholm LH, Black HR, Krum H, Linas S, Linseman JV, Arterburn S, Sager P, Weber M (2010) Divergent results using clinic and ambulatory blood pressures: report of a darusentan-resistant hypertension trial. Hypertension 56(5):824–830
56. Black HR, Bakris GL, Weber MA, Weiss R, Shahawy ME, Marple R, Tannoury G, Linas S, Wiens BL, Linseman JV, Roden R, Gerber MJ (2007) Efficacy and safety of darusentan in patients with resistant hypertension: results from a randomized, double-blind, placebo-controlled dose-ranging study. J Clin Hypertens (Greenwich) 9(10):760–769
57. Symplicity HTN-2 Investigators, Esler MD, Krum H, Sobotka PA, Schlaich MP, Schmieder RE, Böhm M (2010) Renal sympathetic denervation in patients with treatment-resistant hypertension (the simplicity HTN-2 Trial): a randomised controlled trial. Lancet 376(9756):1903–1909

11 The Role of Renal Denervation

Felix Mahfoud and Michael Böhm

11.1 Role of the Renal Sympathetic Nervous System

The sympathetic nervous system innervates the kidneys via efferent fibers from the thoracic and lumbar sympathetic trunks and provides regulation to the central nervous system via afferent (TH10–L4) fibers mediated by stimulation of mechano- and chemoreceptors (Fig. 11.1). The efferent fibers innervate the renal vasculature, the tubular segment of the nephron, and juxtaglomerular renin-containing granular cells [1]. Key events after efferent stimulation of the kidneys are tubular sodium retention (alpha-1B adrenoceptors), reduced renal blood flow (alpha-1A-receptors), and renin release of the juxtaglomerular apparatus (beta-1 adrenoceptors) [1].

11.2 Catheter-Based Renal Denervation

Both the efferent and afferent fibers can be targeted by a catheter-based approach, delivering thermal energy as by radiofrequency. Numerous new percutaneous renal nerve ablation systems are currently being tested and will soon be released into the market. Up to now, the largest experience with the longest clinical follow-ups has been obtained with the Symplicity Catheter System (Medtronic Ardian, Minneapolis, USA). Via a femoral access, a special RF catheter (Symplicity™ Catheter System) is inserted percutaneously and advanced to the distal segment of

F. Mahfoud (✉) · M. Böhm
Klinik für Innere Medizin III, Kardiologie, Angiologie und Internistische Intensivmedizin, Kirrberger Str. 1, Gebäude 40, 66421 Homburg, Saar, Germany
e-mail: felix.mahfoud@uks.eu

M. Böhm
e-mail: Michael.Boehm@uniklinikum-saarland.de

G. Mancia (ed.), *Resistant Hypertension*, DOI: 10.1007/978-88-470-5415-8_11,

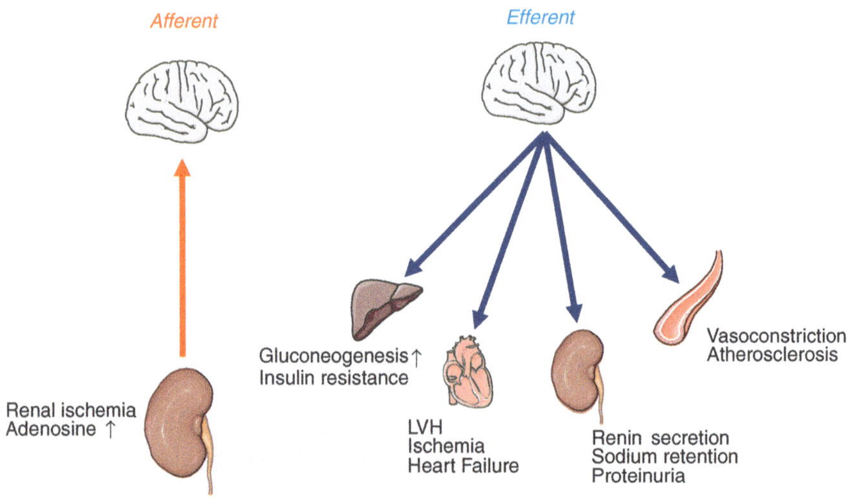

Fig. 11.1 Renal afferent and efferent sympathetic nerves

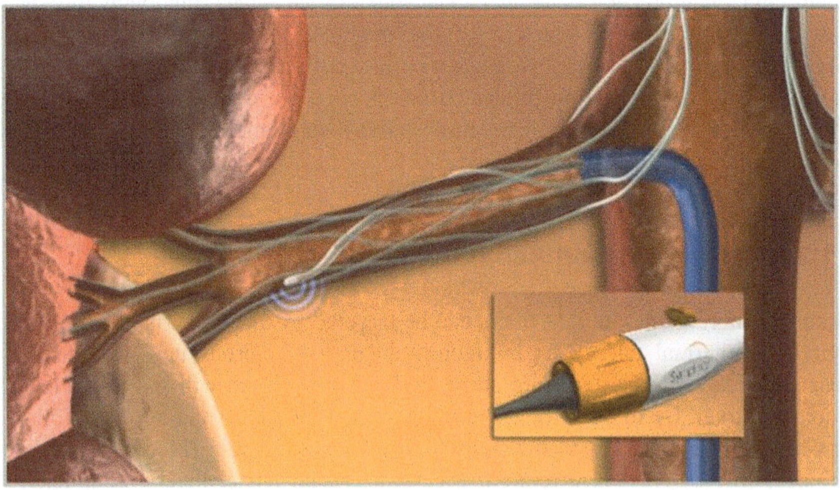

Fig. 11.2 RF ablation using a special catheter placed in the distal segment of the renal artery (courtesy of Medtronic, USA)

the renal artery under fluoroscopy (Fig. 11.2). The vessel wall is focally heated up to a maximum of 70 °C by delivery of radiofrequency energy with a maximum of 8 watts for 120 s. While the vessel is cooled intraluminally by the high renal blood flow, thermal damage is provided to sympathetic nerves located in the adventitia of the renal arteries. Subsequently, the catheter is pulled back from distal to proximal vessel segments, and treatment sites are separated both longitudinally and rotationally with a spacing of >5 mm in order to capture the entire circumference of the vessel. This results in 4–8 ablations per artery depending on its length and circumference. Due to the proximity of sympathetic nerves and C pain fibers, during RF ablation, analgoanesthesia is necessary during the procedure. Heparin is given to achieve an activated clotting time during the procedure of >250 s. In some patients, RF ablations cause renal artery edema/spasm at the treatment sites, which can be treated by intra-arterial injection of nitroglycerin or adenosine. These changes are likely to disappear within hours after treatment.

11.2.1 Clinical Studies

The Symplicity HTN-1 ($n = 45$) published in 2009 was the first multicenter proof-of-concept and safety study for patients with resistant arterial hypertension undergoing catheter-based renal denervation [2]. Patients in the Symplicity HTN-1 study were heavily medicated, taking an average of 4.7 antihypertensive drugs, and were still poorly controlled (office blood pressure 177/101 mmHg). The primary end point was peri-procedural and long-term safety of the treatment. After four weeks, a significant reduction in systolic and diastolic office blood pressures by 14 and 10 mmHg has been described, which increased to 27 and 17 mmHg ($p = 0.026$) after 12 months. The recently presented 36-month long-term follow-up indicates a sustained blood pressure–lowering effect of 33 and 19 mmHg ($p < 0.01$, $n = 24$; Fig. 11.3) [3, 4], making a significant functional regrow or reinnervation of the kidneys unlikely. Antihypertensive background medication was increased in nine patients and decreased in four patients. As secondary end point, a reduction in renal norepinephrine spillover was significantly reduced by 47 % ($n = 10$), providing direct evidence for inhibition of sympathetic activity [2].

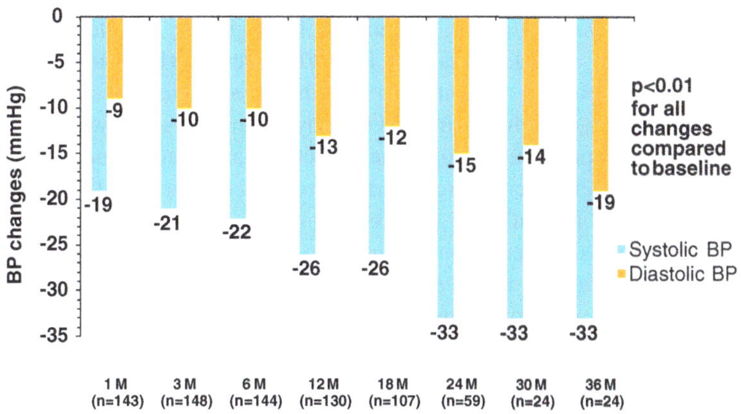

Fig. 11.3 Blood pressure–lowering effect up to 36 months after renal denervation (data from [5])

Consecutively, the multicenter, prospective, randomized Symplicity HTN-2 study included a total of 106 patients with resistant hypertension, randomized 1:1 to a control group (continuation of drug treatment, $n = 54$) and a treatment group (renal denervation plus continued drug treatment, $n = 52$) [3]. Baseline mean office blood pressure was 178/96 mmHg, despite an intake of 5.3 antihypertensive drugs. Six months after renal denervation, mean blood pressure in the treatment group decreased significantly by 32/12 mmHg ($p < 0.0001$) without any changes in the control group. Home-based BP decreased by 20/12 mmHg ($p < 0.0001$, $n = 32$), compared to 2/0 mmHg in the control group ($n = 40$). Reductions in ambulatory blood pressure monitoring over 24 h were lower compared to changes in office-based blood pressure, showing a reduction of 11/7 mmHg in the intervention group ($p = 0.007$, $n = 20$) in contrast to no changes in the control group. Antihypertensive drug regimen was reduced in 10 patients (20 %) within 6 months after renal denervation. Response to treatment was defined as a reduction in SBP > 10 mmHg after 6 months and was found in 84 %. The predictors of response include high systolic baseline blood pressure ($p < 0.001$) and an intake of centrally acting sympatholytics ($p = 0.018$) [2]. At present, no predictors of non-response have been identified.

11.2.2 Safety

Treatments were performed in the Symplicity trials without major complications in 98 % (201/209) of the cases included [2–4]. The following complications have been reported:

- 7 vasovagal reactions (resolved under treatment with atropine)
- 3 femoral artery pseudo-aneurysms
- 1 urinary tract infection
- 1 case of back pain
- 1 extended hospitalization for assessment of paresthesia
- 1 renal artery dissection during placement of the guiding catheter.

Six-month renal vascular imaging in 130 patients who underwent renal denervation identified one patient with possible progression of an underlying atherosclerotic lesion, which required no therapy. It remains unanswered to which extent the ablation procedure and/or the catheter manipulation induced or promoted the rapid development of renal artery stenosis or whether it represented a natural progression of the disease process.

The effect of renal denervation on the physiological response during cardiopulmonary exercise testing has been tested in a sub-study [6]. Renal denervation resulted in a significant drop in resting, maximum exercise, and recovery blood pressure, whereas heart rate response during exercise and oxygen uptake was well preserved (Fig. 11.4).

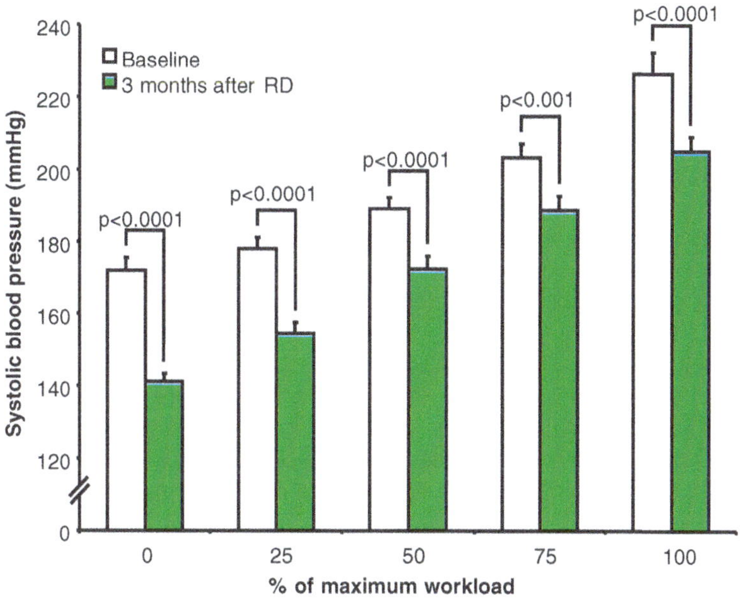

Fig. 11.4 Blood pressure during cardiopulmonary exercise testing before and 3 months after renal denervation (modified with permission from [6])

A recently published study [7] investigated the effect of renal denervation on renal function and urinary albumin excretion in 100 patients with resistant hypertension and preserved renal function. The study demonstrated a reduced number of patients with micro- and macroalbuminuria after renal denervation, without adversely affecting GFR or renal artery structure within six months. It is important to note that in the Symplicity trials, patients with an eGFR < 45 ml/min/1.73 m^2 were excluded as a matter of safety.

11.2.3 Contraindications for Renal Denervation

Several position papers from national and international societies aimed to provide practical recommendations on the application of RDN [8, 9]. The current contraindications for renal denervation are as follows:

- secondary and treatable causes of hypertension
- pseudo-resistant hypertension
- anatomical unsuitability of renal arteries (diameter < 4 mm; length < 20 mm; fibromuscular dysplasia; significant renal artery stenosis; prior renal artery intervention)
- renal insufficiency (GFR < 45 ml/min per 1.73 m^2).

11.2.4 Effects Other than Blood Pressure Lowering

Diabetes Mellitus and Insulin Resistance

Activation of the sympathetic nervous system is a main contributor to insulin resistance, metabolic syndrome, associated with central obesity, and risk of developing diabetes mellitus [10, 11]. A bidirectional relationship between sympathetic overactivity inducing insulin resistance and hyperinsulinemia producing sympathetic activation exists, thus initiating a vicious cycle. In a recently published pilot study [12], renal denervation positively influenced glucose metabolism in patients with resistant hypertension. Three months after the procedure, fasting glucose, fasting insulin, and 2-h glucose concentration during oral glucose tolerance testing were significantly reduced, resulting in a significant improvement in insulin sensitivity (measured using the HOMA Index), whereas there were no changes in the control group (Fig. 11.5). Confirmatory data are coming from a study investigating the effect of renal denervation in patients with obstructive sleep apnea [13]. Beside reductions in the severity of obstructive sleep apnea, the authors report changes in 2-h glucose concentration during oral glucose tolerance test and reductions in HbA1c. A preliminary report in two patients with polycystic ovary syndrome suggests that renal denervation lowers blood pressure and improves insulin resistance (measured by euglycemic clamp methodology) in the absence of changes in body weight over a 3-month period [14]. Further trials are necessary to document the durability of these results as well as their renal, retinal, and cardiovascular consequences in patients suffering from diabetes.

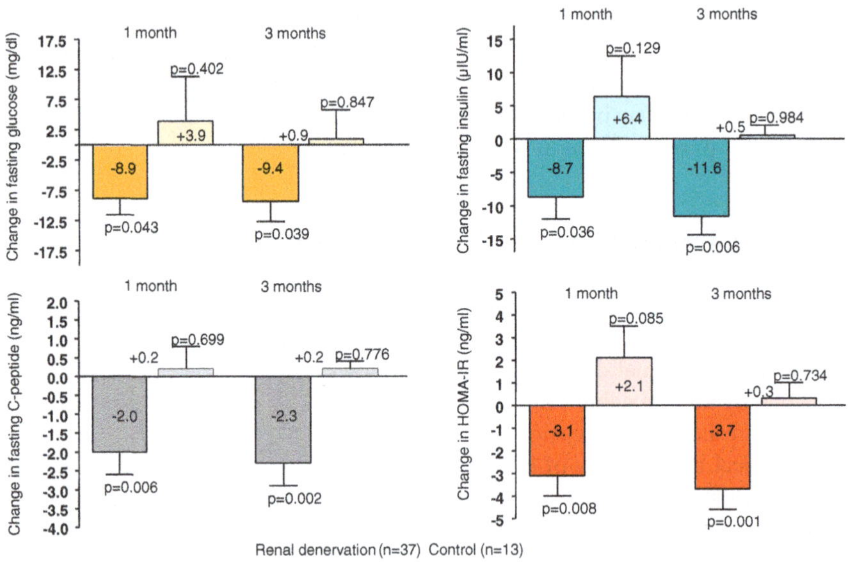

Fig. 11.5 Changes in fasting glucose, insulin, C-peptide, and HOMA Index after renal denervation (modified with permission from [12])

Chronic Heart Failure

Neurohumoral activation, in particular activation of the sympathetic nervous system, is of prognostic relevance in patients with chronic heart failure [15]. The kidneys have been identified as a main contributor to the pathophysiology (i.e., cardiorenal syndrome) [16]. A recently published study investigated the effects of renal denervation on left ventricular mass and diastolic filling pattern in 46 patients with resistant hypertension in which renal denervation was associated with substantial reductions in blood pressure and significantly reduced left ventricular mass and mean interventricular septum thickness [17]. Diastolic function (assessed by mitral valve lateral E/E') was improved after renal denervation, indicating reduction in left ventricular filling pressures, and ejection fraction improved. Interestingly, the changes appeared to be somehow independent of the blood pressure–lowering effects. In a small first-in-man pilot study involving seven, normotensive patients with chronic heart failure undergoing renal denervation six months after treatment, 6-min walk distance significantly increased and patients' self-assessment improved [18]. There were no significant changes in blood pressure, renal function, and no symptomatic fluctuations in hemodynamics. A randomized, controlled multicenter trial investigating the effects of renal denervation in 100 patients with chronic heart failure in NYHA functional class II–III is currently conducted and will provide important information.

Chronic Kidney Disease

Abundant evidence shows that chronic kidney disease is characterized by sympathetic activation, contributing to hypertension and the progressive loss of renal function [19]. Renal denervation could therefore be a potentially novel therapeutic strategy in patients with impaired renal function, including end-stage kidney disease. However, as in the Symplicity trials, patients with a GFR < 45 ml/min/1.73 m^2 were excluded as the safety of such an intervention in this patient population is uncertain. Recently, the effects of renal denervation in a small series of 15 patients with moderate-to-severe chronic kidney disease (mean GFR 31 ml/min/1.73 m^2) were reported [20]. Renal denervation was equally effective in terms of blood pressure lowering, and there was no evidence of a further decline in GFR or effective renal plasma flow 6 months after the procedure, despite exposure to contrast medium. Due to the limited data, however, patients with higher grades of renal insufficiency should only be treated in the context of scientific protocols.

Antiarrhythmic Effects

The autonomic nervous system also modulates cardiac electrophysiological properties including chronotropy and dromotropy, depolarization rate of the sinus node, and atrioventricular conduction [21]. Indeed, renal denervation significantly lowered resting heart rate in patients with resistant hypertension and prolonged PR interval [22]. Interestingly, neither baseline heart rate nor changes in heart rate correlated with the blood pressure reductions. In a first-in-human experience, renal denervation was used as bailout therapy in two patients with congestive heart failure suffering from treatment-resistant electrical storm [23]. Following renal denervation, ventricular tachyarrhythmias were significantly reduced in both patients. The impact of renal denervation in patients with refractory atrial fibrillation and resistant hypertension has been assessed in a recently published study [24]. Twenty-seven patients were randomized to pulmonary vein isolation alone or pulmonary vein isolation plus renal denervation. Besides significant reductions in blood pressure, patients in the pulmonary vein isolation plus renal denervation group experienced significantly fewer episodes of atrial fibrillation at follow-up. Furthermore, animal experiments support the antiarrhythmic effects of renal denervation and suggest a reduced inducibility of atrial fibrillation after the procedure [25].

11.3 Outlook

Currently, the multicenter, prospective, single-blind, randomized, and placebo-controlled Symplicity HTN-3 study (NCT01418261) is ongoing and will hopefully answer the question of a contributing placebo effects after renal denervation. In order to assess the long-term effects of treatment, an international registry (Symplicity Global Registry; NCT01534299) has been conducted to facilitate a systematic follow-up of >5,000 patients undergoing renal denervation in >250 sites. Trials including patients with mild-to-moderate forms of hypertension will be important to definitely assess the role of renal denervation in antihypertensive treatment.

References

1. DiBona GF (2005) Physiology in perspective: the wisdom of the body. Neural control of the kidney. Am J Physiol Regul Integr Comp Physiol 289(3):R633–641
2. Krum H, Schlaich M, Whitbourn R, Sobotka PA, Sadowski J, Bartus K, Kapelak B, Walton A, Sievert H, Thambar S, Abraham WT, Esler M (2009) Catheter-based renal sympathetic denervation for resistant hypertension: a multicentre safety and proof-of-principle cohort study. Lancet 373(9671):1275–1281
3. Esler MD, Krum H, Sobotka PA, Schlaich MP, Schmieder RE, Böhm M (2010) Renal sympathetic denervation in patients with treatment-resistant hypertension (The Symplicity HTN-2 Trial): a randomised controlled trial. Lancet 376(9756):1903–1909
4. Krum H, Barman N, Schlaich M, Sobotka P, Esler M, Mahfoud F, Böhm M, Dunlap M (2011) Catheter-based renal sympathetic denervation for resistant hypertension: durability of blood pressure reduction out to 24 months. Hypertension 57(5):911–917
5. Krum H, Barman N, Schlaich M, Sobotka P, Esler M, Mahfoud F (2012) Long-term follow-up of catheter-based renal sympathetic denervation for resistant hypertension confirms durable blood pressure reduction. J Am Coll Cardiol 59:E1705
6. Ukena C, Mahfoud F, Kindermann I, Barth C, Lenski M, Kindermann M, Brandt MC, Hoppe UC, Krum H, Esler M, Sobotka PA, Böhm M (2011) Cardiorespiratory response to exercise after renal sympathetic denervation in patients with resistant hypertension. J Am Coll Cardiol 58(11):1176–1182

7. Mahfoud F, Cremers B, Janker J, Link B, Vonend O, Ukena C, Linz D, Schmieder R, Rump LC, Kindermann I, Sobotka PA, Krum H, Scheller B, Schlaich M, Laufs U, Böhm M (2012) Renal hemodynamics and renal function after catheter-based renal sympathetic denervation in patients with resistant hypertension. Hypertension 60(2):419–424
8. Mahfoud F, Vonend O, Bruck H, Clasen W, Eckert S, Frye B, Haller H, Hausberg M, Hoppe UC, Hoyer J, Hahn K, Keller T, Krämer BK, Kreutz R, Potthoff SA, Reinecke H, Schmieder R, Schwenger V, Kintscher U, Böhm M, Rump LC (2011) Expert consensus statement on interventional renal sympathetic denervation for hypertension treatment. Dtsch Med Wochenschr 136(47):2418
9. Schmieder RE, Redon J, Grassi G, Kjeldsen SE, Mancia G, Narkiewicz K, Parati G, Ruilope L, van de Borne P, Tsioufis C (2012) ESH position paper: renal denervation—an interventional therapy of resistant hypertension. J Hypertens 30(5):837–841
10. Grassi G, Dell'Oro R, Quarti-Trevano F, Scopelliti F, Seravalle G, Paleari F, Gamba PL, Mancia G (2005) Neuroadrenergic and reflex abnormalities in patients with metabolic syndrome. Diabetologia 48(7):1359–1365
11. Huggett RJ, Scott EM, Gilbey SG, Stoker JB, Mackintosh AF, Mary DA (2003) Impact of type 2 diabetes mellitus on sympathetic neural mechanisms in hypertension. Circulation 108(25):3097–3101
12. Mahfoud F, Schlaich M, Kindermann I, Ukena C, Cremers B, Brandt MC, Hoppe UC, Vonend O, Rump LC, Sobotka PA, Krum H, Esler M, Böhm M (2011) Effect of renal sympathetic denervation on glucose metabolism in patients with resistant hypertension: a pilot study. Circulation 123(18):1940–1946
13. Witkowski A, Prejbisz A, Florczak E, Kadziela J, Sliwinski P, Bielen P, Michalowska I, Kabat M, Warchol E, Januszewicz M, Narkiewicz K, Somers VK, Sobotka PA, Januszewicz A (2011) Effects of renal sympathetic denervation on blood pressure, sleep apnea course, and glycemic control in patients with resistant hypertension and sleep apnea. Hypertension 58(4):559–565
14. Schlaich MP, Straznicky N, Grima M, Ika-Sari C, Dawood T, Mahfoud F, Lambert E, Chopra R, Socratous F, Hennebry S, Eikelis N, Böhm M, Krum H, Lambert G, Esler MD, Sobotka PA (2011) Renal denervation: a potential new treatment modality for polycystic ovary syndrome? J Hypertens 29(5):991–996
15. Parati G, Esler M (2012) The human sympathetic nervous system: its relevance in hypertension and heart failure. Eur Heart J 33(9):1058–1066
16. Rundqvist B, Elam M, Bergmann-Sverrisdottir Y, Eisenhofer G, Friberg P (1997) Increased cardiac adrenergic drive precedes generalized sympathetic activation in human heart failure. Circulation 95(1):169–175
17. Brandt MC, Mahfoud F, Reda S, Schirmer SH, Erdmann E, Böhm M, Hoppe UC (2012) Renal sympathetic denervation reduces left ventricular hypertrophy and improves cardiac function in patients with resistant hypertension. J Am Coll Cardiol 59(10):901–909
18. Davies JE, Manisty CH, Petraco R, Barron AJ, Unsworth B, Mayet J, Hamady M, Hughes AD, Sever PS, Sobotka PA, Francis DP (2012) First-in-man safety evaluation of renal denervation for chronic systolic heart failure: Primary outcome from REACH-Pilot study. Int J Cardiol 2012, online, in press
19. Schlaich MP, Socratous F, Hennebry S, Eikelis N, Lambert EA, Straznicky N, Esler MD, Lambert GW (2009) Sympathetic activation in chronic renal failure. J Am Soc Nephrol 20(5):933–939
20. Hering D, Mahfoud F, Walton AS, Krum H, Lambert GW, Lambert EA, Sobotka PA, Böhm M, Cremers B, Esler MD, Schlaich MP (2012) Renal denervation in moderate to severe CKD. J Am Soc Nephrol 23(7):1250–1257
21. Inoue H, Zipes DP (1987) Changes in atrial and ventricular refractoriness and in atrioventricular nodal conduction produced by combinations of vagal and sympathetic stimulation that result in a constant spontaneous sinus cycle length. Circ Res 60(6):942–951

22. Ukena C, Mahfoud F, Spies A, Kindermann I, Linz D, Cremers B, Laufs U, Neuberger HR, Böhm M (2012) Effects of renal sympathetic denervation on heart rate and atrioventricular conduction in patients with resistant hypertension. Int J Cardiol 2012, online, in press
23. Ukena C, Bauer A, Mahfoud F, Schreieck J, Neuberger HR, Eick C, Sobotka PA, Gawaz M, Böhm M (2012) Renal sympathetic denervation for treatment of electrical storm: first-in-man experience. Clin Res Cardiol 101(1):63–67
24. Pokushalov E, Romanov A, Corbucci G, Artyomenko S, Baranova V, Turov A, Shirokova N, Karaskov A, Mittal S, Steinberg JS (2012) A randomized comparison of pulmonary vein isolation with versus without concomitant renal artery denervation in patients with refractory symptomatic atrial fibrillation and resistant hypertension. J Am Coll Cardiol 60(13): 1163–1170
25. Linz D, Mahfoud F, Schotten U, Ukena C, Neuberger HR, Wirth K, Böhm M (2012) Renal sympathetic denervation suppresses postapneic blood pressure rises and atrial fibrillation in a model for sleep apnea. Hypertension 60(1):172–178

12 The Role of Carotid Baroreceptor Stimulation

Guido Grassi, Gianmaria Brambilla and Gino Seravalle

12.1 Introduction

Along with the renal nerve ablation approach, which has been already examined in detail in the previous chapter of this book, another invasive procedure based on stimulation of arterial baroreceptors located within the wall of the carotid arteries (carotid sinuses), known as electrical carotid baroreceptor stimulation, has received in the past few years particular interest for the treatment of resistant hypertension. This chapter will be focused on this approach, examining in sequence (1) the rationale for this intervention, (2) its historical background and main features, and (3) the results so far obtained in the field of resistant hypertension. The chapter will also provide, in its final part, a critical evaluation of the approach, with an analysis of its potential main advantages and disadvantages as compared with the renal denervation approach.

12.2 Rationale for the Carotid Baroreceptor Stimulation Approach

Three main sets of information represent the background for the procedure based on the electrical stimulation of the carotid baroreceptors via programmable impulse generator devices. The first one refers to the notion that receptors located

G. Grassi (✉) · G. Brambilla
Clinica Medica, University of Milano-Bicocca, Ospedale S.Gerardo dei Tintori
Via Pergolesi 33, 20052 Monza, MI, Italy

Istituto di Ricerca e Cura a Carattere Scientifico Multimedica, Sesto San Giovanni, MI, Italy
e-mail: guido.grassi@unimib.it

G. Seravalle
Istituto Auxologico Italiano, Via Dominichino, 22148 Italiano, MI, Italy

G. Mancia (ed.), *Resistant Hypertension*, DOI: 10.1007/978-88-470-5415-8_12,

in the transverse aortic arch (aortic baroreceptors) as well as in the carotid sinuses of the left and right internal carotid arteries (carotid baroreceptors), known under the term of "arterial baroreceptors," exert an important regulatory function in the homeostatic control of blood pressure, by controlling a number of cardiovascular parameters (Table 12.1) [1]. Arterial baroreceptors are stretch receptors that are stimulated by distortion of the arterial wall when pressure changes. The baroreceptors can recognize the changes in both the average blood pressure or the rate of change in pressure with each arterial pulse. Action potentials triggered in the baroreceptor endings are then conducted to the brainstem transmitting this information to neurons within the central nervous system [1]. In man, stimulation or deactivation of arterial baroreceptors can be achieved by a variety of techniques, such as infusion in the systemic circulation of vasoactive drugs (phenylephrine or nitroprusside) or the application of positive or negative pressures within a device positioned at the level of the neck, where carotid arteries and carotid baroreceptors are anatomically located [1]. By using these techniques, it has been possible to show that in physiological conditions in which blood pressure increases, there is a marked deactivation of aortic and carotid baroreceptors. This triggers a decrease in heart rate and an inhibition of sympathetic vasoconstrictor drive. As a net result, blood pressure decreases with a concomitant reduction in cardiac output and in peripheral vascular resistance. Conversely, in physiological conditions in which blood pressure decreases, there is a marked stimulation of aortic and carotid baroreceptors. This triggers an increase in heart rate and an enhancement of sympathetic vasoconstrictor drive. As a net result, blood pressure increases with a concomitant raise in cardiac output and in peripheral vascular resistance.

The second notion, on the other hand, refers to the evidence that arterial baroreceptor (and particularly carotid baroreceptor) function is impaired in essential hypertension [1, 2]. This baroreceptor dysfunction includes on one hand the impairment of baroreceptor modulation of heart rate (which is mediated by vagal fibers) and on the other by an alteration in the baroreceptor control of blood pressure (which is mediated by and sympathetic fibers) (Fig. 12.1). In this latter case, as it will be discussed below, the baroreceptor alteration is known as "resetting" of the operational set point of the reflex function [2]. In practical

Table 12.1 Cardiovascular effects of alterations in carotid baroreceptor activity

Variable	Baroreceptor stimulation	Baroreceptor deactivation
Heart rate	Reduced	Increased
Atrioventricular conduction time	Increased	Reduced
Cardiac output	Slightly reduced	Slightly increased
Peripheral resistance	Reduced	Increased
Splanchnic circulation	Vasodilation	Vasoconstriction
Muscle circulation	No change	No change

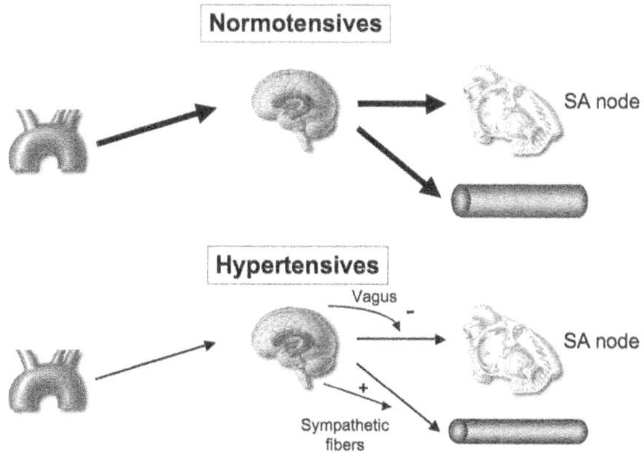

Fig. 12.1 Scheme illustrating the normal control of heart rate and peripheral vessels exerted by carotid baroreceptors in the normotensive state (*upper panel*) and its alterations in hypertension (*lower panel*). These cause a reduction (−) in vagal control of the heart and a potentiation (+) in sympathetic vasoconstrictor tone. *SA* sinus node activity

terms, this means that, although not primarily altered, baroreceptor control of blood pressure is reset toward more elevated blood pressure values with an attenuation of its pressor influences and a potentiation of the depressor ones.

A third and final notion should be discussed when considering the pathophysiological background of the procedure based on the electrical stimulation of the carotid baroreceptors, that is, the fact that essential hypertension is a clinical condition characterized by a marked sympathetic stimulation (Fig. 12.2) [3, 4], brought about by a variety of factors including the arterial baroreceptor impairment. Because this adrenergic overdrive has a number of adverse effects on blood pressure, cardiovascular homeostasis as well as on metabolic function, it represents an important target of the non-pharmacological as well as of the pharmacological interventions aimed at reducing elevated blood pressure values [3, 4].

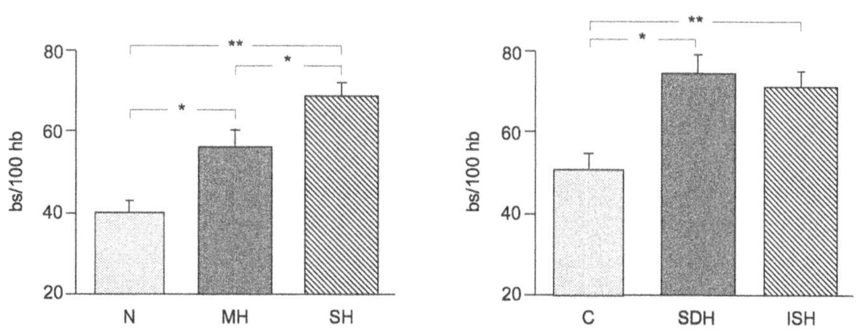

Fig. 12.2 Values of muscle sympathetic nerve traffic, measured via the microneurographic technique, in normotensive control subjects (*N* and *C*) and in patients with mild hypertension (*MH*), severe hypertension (*SH*), systodiastolic hypertension (*SDH*), and isolated systolic hypertension (*ISH*). Data are shown as means ± standard error. From data included in [4, 5]

This is the case also for the renal nerves ablation approach and for the electrical stimulation of the carotid baroreceptors, because both the interventions have been shown to exert sustained sympathoinhibitory effects [5].

12.3 Results of Studies in Experimental Animal Models

The goal of lowering blood pressure in humans by activating carotid baroreceptors is not a new approach. The first studies performed in experimental animals about 60 years ago showed that a significant reduction in blood pressure was achieved in normotensive or hypertensive dogs for several hours following direct electrical stimulation of the carotid sinus nerve [6–8]. In the first years of the millennium, studies by different investigators showed that, in animals with angiotensin II-induced acute and chronic hypertension, this treatment produced a decrease in renal sympathetic nerve activity in animals with an intact baroreflex but not in animals that had undergone sinoaortic denervation [9–11]. These data suggest that the baroreflex is important in chronic hypertension and that renal sympathoinhibition, with a resultant increase in natriuresis, may be the mechanism by which the baroreflex participates in long-term blood pressure control [9, 12]. A further step was evaluation of the effects of the long-term stimulation of the baroreflex using electrodes implanted around both carotid sinuses of dogs [13]. Baroreflex activation for 7 days elicited a rapid and sustained reduction in heart rate and blood pressure as well as a significant reduction in plasma levels of the adrenergic neurotransmitter norepinephrine. More recently, the same group of authors evaluated the effects of prolonged electrical carotid baroreflex stimulation in dogs with obesity-induced hypertension, showing a significant reduction in mean arterial pressure and plasma catecholamines without a concomitant increase in plasma renin activity [13]. Thus, in obesity, baroreflex activation can suppress the endogenous activation of the sympathetic nervous system and reduce high blood pressure. These data also support the hypothesis that baroreflex-mediated suppression of renal sympathetic nerve activity is an important mechanism by which the carotid stimulation exerts its antihypertensive effect.

12.4 Results of Clinical Studies and Clinical Trials

The hemodynamic effects of bilateral electrical stimulation of the carotid sinus nerves in humans have been evaluated in several studies. In one study [14], the acute carotid stimulation of supine hypertensive patients reduced cardiac output by 11 %, peripheral resistance by 10 %, mean arterial pressure by 21 %, and heart rate by 16 %. Similar results were also reported in other studies [15, 16].

Following this earlier experience, the development of systems that permitted radiofrequency adjustment of implanted devices allowed in the earlier 1960s to better tailor stimulation of parameters to individual patients. In recent years, the availability of a programmable impulse generator (positioned in a subcutaneous pocket at the level of the chest) allowed the intermittent stimulation of the baroreceptors (frequency: 20–100 Hz; amplitude: 4.0–7.0 V) through two active electrodes implanted with neck surgery at the level of the left and right carotid sinuses [17]. Clinical experience with the device has been collected so far in a small number of clinical studies and trials whose main results can be summarized as follows. The first data were collected in the Rheos Feasibility Trial, with an acronym that refers to the surgically implantable device (Rheos System; CVRx Inc., Minneapolis, MN, USA) tested in a study monitored by the United States Food and Drug Administration [18]. The trial was carried out in ten patients with resistant hypertension taking on average six antihypertensive drugs without achieving effective blood pressure control. Following a recovery time after implantation of one month, the device was activated, and this enabled a marked blood pressure reduction with a maximal response amounting to 42 mmHg for systolic and 21 mmHg for diastolic blood pressure. The magnitude of the response was quite stable over the follow-up of the study (10 months), although the rough data were not included in this first publication. Apart from two cases of infections at the level of the surgical intervention, which were treated successfully, the procedure was uneventful and without significant side effects. This initial publication was followed by two other papers aimed at clarifying the mechanisms through which the procedure was capable of reducing blood pressure [19, 20]. Both these studies confirmed the profound sympathoinhibition triggered by the electric field stimulation of carotid baroreceptors, the magnitude of which was directly and significantly related to the degree of the systolic blood pressure reduction elicited by the intervention. Other remarkable effects of the procedure were represented by (1) a small heart rate reduction, (2) a decrease in plasma renin activity levels (about 20 %), (3) a tendency of heart rate variability to increase in the low-frequency component (an index of improvement in vagal control of the heart), and (4) a substantially unchanged baroreflex modulation of heart rate, as dynamically assessed via cross-spectral analysis and sequence technique. In one of these studies [21], the blood pressure-lowering effects of the intervention were documented not only via classic sphygmomanometric blood pressure measurements but also via 24-h ambulatory monitoring, thereby providing information on a variable such as daily-life blood pressure that has a special importance for the patient's prognosis [22]. The magnitude of the 24-h blood pressure reduction (on average 10 mmHg for systolic and 6 mmHg for diastolic blood pressure) only seems small if one takes into account that drug treatment–induced changes in 24-h mean blood pressure are usually much smaller than the corresponding changes in clinic blood pressure [23]. The information collected in these earlier studies was supplemented by the results of 2 recent trials, the Device-Based Therapy in Hypertension Trial (DEBuT-HT) [24] and the Rheos Pivotal Trial [24], enrolling 45 and 265 patients with resistant hypertension, respectively. Their results can be summarized as follows. First, the sustained effectiveness of the procedure was confirmed over the long term, with evidence that at two years of follow-up, stimulation of carotid baroreceptors retained the blood pressure-lowering effects seen in the earlier period. Second, about 20 % of patients experienced side effects, which were mostly directly related to the surgical or anesthetic procedure (local surgical complications, nerve injury, etc.). Finally, about half of the implanted patients achieved at the 6-month follow-up, systolic blood pressure control allowing them to substantially reduce both the number and the daily dosage of the antihypertensive drugs unsuccessfully used prior to the procedure. Technical refinements to the methodological approach as well as the surgical procedure will enable in the next years a less invasive approach to be used, based on a single electrode positioned only on one side of the neck and thus performing a monolateral carotid baroreceptor stimulation. Preliminary experience with the new approach has indeed shown that it allows the coupling of efficacy with an improved side effect profile [5].

12.5 Electrical Stimulation of Carotid Baroreceptors Versus Renal Denervation

Our group has recently made a vis-a-vis comparison of the results of the two procedures available for lowering blood pressure in resistant hypertension [5]. The results of this analysis can be summarized as follows. First, both the two techniques have been shown to reduce in short-term and in the medium-term period (3–4 years) clinic blood pressure values, while less information is available,

		Renal Denervation	Carotid Baroreceptor Stimulation
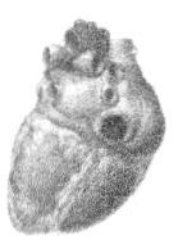	LV diastolic function	↑↑	-
	LV mass index	↓↓	↓
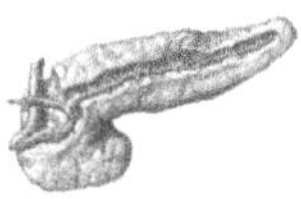	Fasting glucose levels	↓	?
	HOMA-IR	↓	?
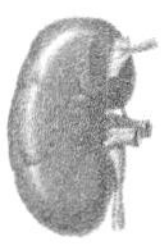	eGFR	=	=
	Microalbuminuria	↓	?

Fig. 12.3 Scheme illustrating the effects of renal denervation and electrical stimulation of carotid baroreceptors on hypertension-related end-organ damage. *LV* left ventricular, *HOMA-IR* homeostasis model assessment of insulin resistance, *eGFR* estimated glomerular filtration rate. ↑↑ improvement, ↓ reduction, = no change,? effect unknown

particularly for renal denervation, for ambulatory blood pressure. The data so far obtained, however, show a 24-h ambulatory blood pressure reduction less marked than the clinic one. In contrast, there are a number of studies which have assessed the impact of renal denervation on both organ damage and metabolic alterations accompanying resistant hypertension (Fig. 12.3). Several of these information, however, are still lacking in the case of electrical stimulation of the carotid baroreceptors (Fig. 12.3). Finally, an analysis of potential clinical complications associated with the interventions indicates the greater safety (and the reduced side effects profile) of the renal denervation approach as compared to the baroreceptor stimulation method, which requires a surgical intervention.

12.6 Conclusions

Although intriguing, the results obtained via the procedure based on electrical stimulation of the carotid baroreceptors for the treatment of resistant hypertension leave open a number of clinically relevant questions. These will call for new investigations on this procedure, which nevertheless represents a new therapeutic options for this condition.

References

1. Mancia G, Mark AL (1983) Arterial baroreflexes in humans. In: Shepherd JT, Abboud EM (eds) Handbook of physiology, section 2: the cardiovascular system. American Physiological Society, Bethesda, MD, pp 755–793
2. Mancia G, Ludbrook J, Ferrari A et al (1978) Baroreceptor reflexes in human hypertension. Circ Res 43:170–177
3. Grassi G (2009) Assessment of sympathetic cardiovascular drive in human hypertension: achievements and perspectives. Hypertension 54:690–697
4. Grassi G (2010) Sympathetic neural activity in hypertension and related diseases. Am J Hypertens 23:1052–1058
5. Grassi G, Seravalle G, Brambilla G et al (2012) Novel antihypertensive therapies: renal sympathetic nerve ablation and carotid baroreceptor stimulation. Curr Hypertens Rep 14:567–572
6. McCubbin JW, Green JH, Page IH (1956) Baroreceptor function in chronic renal hypertension. Circ Res 4:205–210
7. Werner HR (1958) The frequency-dependent nature of blood pressure regulation by the carotid sinus studied with an electrical analog. Circ Res 6:35–40
8. Bilgutay A, Lillehei W (1965) Treatment of hypertension with an implantable electronic device. JAMA 191:113–117
9. Lohmeier TE, Loheimer JR, Haque A et al (2000) Baroreflexes prevent neurally induced sodium retention in angiotensin hypertension. Am J Physiol Regul Integr Comp Physiol 279:R1437–R1448
10. Lohmeier TE, Irwin E, Rossing M et al (2004) Prolonged activation of the baroreflex produces sustained hypotension. Hypertension 44:306–311
11. Barrett CJ, Guild S, Ramchandra J et al (2005) Baroreceptor denervation prevents sympathoinhibition during angiotensin II-induced hypertension. Hypertension 46:1–5

12. Lohmeier TE, Hildebrandt DA, Warren S et al (2005) Recent insights into the interactions between the baroreflex and the kidneys in hypertension. Am J Physiol Regul Integr Comp Physiol 288:R828–R836
13. Lohmeier TE, Dwyer TM, Irwin ED et al (2007) Prolonged activation of the baroreflex abolishes obesity-induced hypertension. Hypertension 49:1307–1314
14. Schwartz S, Griffith L, Neistadt A et al (1967) Chronic carotid sinus nerve stimulation in the treatment of essential hypertension. Am J Surg 114:5–15
15. Tuckman J, Reich T, Lyon A et al (1972) Evaluation of carotid sinus nerve stimulation in the treatment of hypertension. Ther Umsch 29:382–391
16. Peters T, Koralewski H, Zerbst F (1989) Search for optimal frequencies and amplitudes of therapeutic electrical carotid sinus nerve stimulation by application of the evolutionary strategy. Artif Organs 13:133–143
17. Lohmeier TE, Dwyer TM, Irwin ED et al (2007) Prolonged activation of the baroreflex abolishes obesity-induced hypertension. Hypertension 49:1307–1314
18. Illig KA, Levy M, Sanchez L et al (2006) An implantable carotid sinus stimulator for drug-resistant hypertension: surgical technique and short-term outcome from the multicenter phase II Rheos feasibility trial. J Vasc Surg 44:1213–1218
19. Wustmann K, Kucera JP, Scheffers I et al (2009) Effects of chronic baroreceptor stimulation on the autonomic cardiovascular regulation in patients with drug-resistant arterial hypertension. Hypertension 54:530–536
20. Heusser K, Tank J, Engeli S et al (2010) Carotid baroreceptor stimulation, sympathetic activity, baroreflex function, and blood pressure in hypertensive patients. Hypertension 55:619–626
21. Sega R, Facchetti R, Bombelli M et al (2005) Prognostic value of ambulatory and home blood pressures compared with office blood pressure in the general population: follow-up results from the Pressioni Arteriose Monitorate e Loro Associazioni (PAMELA) study. Circulation 111:1777–1783
22. Mancia G, Parati G (2004) Office compared with ambulatory blood pressure in assessing response to antihypertensive treatment: a meta-analysis. J Hypertens 22:435–445
23. Scheffers IJ, Kroon AA, Schmidli J et al (2009) Novel baroreflex activation therapy in resistant hypertension: results of a European multi-center feasibility study. J Am Coll Cardiol 56:1254–1258
24. Bisognano JD, Bakris G, Nadim MK et al (2011) Baroreflex activation therapy lowers blood pressure in patients with resistant hypertension: results from the double-blind, randomized, placebo-controlled Rheos pivotal trial. J Am Coll Cardiol 58:765–773

Pathophysiology: Metabolic Alterations and Risk Factors

13

Peter M. Nilsson and Jan Cederholm

13.1 Introduction

Resistant hypertension is a condition that is associated not only with difficult-to-treat hypertension but also with a number of other concomitant cardiovascular risk factors. For example, there are several metabolic abnormalities that have been linked to resistant hypertension, even when secondary hypertension has been excluded with its many examples of endocrine disturbances, that is, acromegaly (GH increase), Mb Cushing (hypercortisolism), or pheochromocytoma (increased catecholamines), where disturbed glucose metabolism and impaired insulin sensitivity is often found. The overall prevalence of resistant hypertension is supposed to be around 12–15 %.

One early observation from a population-based study in Sweden was that patients with refractory (resistant) hypertension often exhibited signs of insulin resistance and the typical metabolic abnormalities linked with this, most importantly hyperglycemia and dyslipidemia (high triglycerides and low HDL cholesterol levels) [1, 2]. In one of the studies, male subjects were further investigated by biopsies of *Musculus vastus lateralis* since structural conditions in skeletal muscles might play a role in this association. Irrespective of pre-study drug therapy, these therapy-resistant hypertensives had a lower insulin sensitivity index than controls ($p < 0.05$). In spite of the BMI-matching, the waist/hip ratio (WHR) in the males with resistant hypertension tended to be higher ($p < 0.07$). Insulin

---

P. M. Nilsson (✉)
Department of Clinical Sciences, Lund University, Skåne University Hospital,
S-205 02 Malmö, Sweden
e-mail: Peter.Nilsson@med.lu.se

J. Cederholm
Department of Public Health and Caring Sciences/Family Medicine and Preventive
Medicine, Uppsala University, S-751 85 Uppsala, Sweden
e-mail: jan.cederholm@pubcare.uu.se

G. Mancia (ed.), *Resistant Hypertension*, DOI: 10.1007/978-88-470-5415-8_13,

clearance tended to be lower in these subjects ($p = 0.09$), and BMI correlated with a reduced muscular capillary density ($r = -0.77$, $p < 0.01$). The average cross-sectional muscle fiber area was larger in RH subjects ($p < 0.05$). Furthermore, the mean muscle fiber area correlated with basal serum insulin ($r = 0.63$; $p < 0.05$). Rarefaction of the muscular capillary bed appears to be related to obesity. Larger muscle fibers might be an effect of the growth factor properties of insulin itself and could possibly correspond to hypertrophy of smooth muscle in the resistance vessels. This factor might contribute to the association of hyperinsulinemia with essential hypertension and attenuate the response to antihypertensive therapy, as shown in patients with resistant hypertension [2].

Another clinical feature of these patients was widespread muscular tension and painful symptoms but also nervous complaints and mental distress, as well as an increased burden of psychosocial stress [3]. The prognosis of resistant hypertension so far in these patients has often been poor due to insufficient treatment of hypertension and the concomitant cardiovascular risk factors [4]. The conclusion is therefore that the total cardiovascular risk profile should be evaluated and targeted in these patients, not only the difficult-to-treat blood pressure.

13.2 Large Register Studies from Spain

Other studies have shown similar characteristics of patients with resistant hypertension from the population. In particular, studies from Spanish populations have documented the high prevalence of obesity, metabolic syndrome, and target organ damage in resistant hypertensive subjects [5–7]. In one screening study, 513 patients were included (64 ± 11 years old, 47 % women). Central obesity was present in 65.7 % (CI 95 % 61.6–69.9), 38.6 % (CI 95 % 34.4–42.8) had diabetes, and 63.7 % (CI 95 % 59.4–67.9) had features indicating the metabolic syndrome. The prevalence of left ventricular hypertrophy and left atrial enlargement determined by echocardiography was 57.1 % (CI 95 % 50.8–63.5) and 10.0 % (CI 95 % 6.3–13.7), respectively. Microalbuminuria was found in 46.6 % (CI 95 % 41.4–51.8) of the subjects. Patients with metabolic syndrome were significantly older (65.4 ± 11 and 62.5 ± 12 years; $P = 0.0052$), presented a higher prevalence of diabetes (52.0 % vs. 16.6; $P < 0.0001$), and were treated more frequently with ≥4 antihypertensive drugs (65.1 vs. 50.0 %, $P = 0.011$). The authors thus concluded that the prevalence of central obesity, metabolic syndrome, and target organ damage is very high in resistant hypertensive subjects [5]. This study should preferably be repeated in other countries and populations at varying cardiovascular risk.

Based on the Spanish register data, resistant hypertension is present in 12 % of the treated hypertensive population, but among them more than one-third have normal ambulatory blood pressure. A worse risk profile in general is associated with true resistant hypertension, but this association is weak, thus making it necessary to assess ambulatory blood pressure monitoring for a correct diagnosis and management.

13.3 Obstructive Sleep Apnea Syndrome

The hemodynamic and metabolic abnormalities linked to resistant hypertension are also prevalent in obesity complicated with obstructive sleep apnea (OSA) syndrome, influencing disturbed sleep patterns and increased nocturnal sympathetic nervous activation. This has been shown in several epidemiological studies and further described in a recent European position paper [8]. One important contributing factor might be chronic inflammation, for example, elevation of TNF-alpha in patients with hypertension and OSA [9]. In particular, in family practice, it is important to recognize resistant hypertension [10] but also to detect and treat OSA, for later referral for continuous positive airway pressure (CPAP) treatment at hospital centers.

13.4 Hyperaldosteronism and the Metabolic Syndrome

A new aspect of this risk factor constellation is the finding that high levels of serum aldosterone are often linked to insulin resistance and metabolic abnormalities as well as elevated blood pressure. Sometimes, a thorough investigation might reveal the existence of secondary hypertension based on the existence of, for example, adrenal adenoma (Conn's syndrome). However, also within the normal or near normal range of aldosteronism, there is reason to believe that this factor could play an important role for the constellation of cardiovascular risk factors so often associated with the metabolic syndrome and resistant hypertension [11, 12]. Accumulating evidence indicates that the cardiovascular and renal abnormalities associated with insulin resistance are mediated, in part, by aldosterone's non-genomic as well as genomic signaling through the mineralocorticoid receptor (MR). In the so-called cardio-metabolic syndrome, there are often increased circulating levels of glucocorticoids, which can also activate MR signaling in cardiovascular, adipose, skeletal muscle, neuronal, and liver tissue. Furthermore, there is increasing evidence that fat tissue produces a lipid-soluble factor that stimulates aldosterone production from the adrenal *zona glomerulosa*, according to one review [12]. These findings should encourage research activities on pathophysiology but also to investigate metabolic and hemodynamic effects following the blockade of aldosterone by use of antagonists. Both older and newer drugs could be used for blocking the aldosterone system, so far with proven benefits in congestive heart failure but not well documented in essential hypertension.

13.5 Endocrine Abnormalities and Disturbed Autonomic Nervous Function

Abnormalities of the autonomous nervous system represent another facet of this risk cluster, often linked to insulin resistance and other features of the metabolic syndrome [13]. Type 2 diabetes is generally associated with greater autonomic imbalance, lower adiponectin levels, and greater BMI in patients with resistant hypertension [13]. It has even been shown that renal nerve ablation has improved not only resistant hypertension but also some of the metabolic abnormalities linked to this condition, for example, impaired glucose metabolism in a pilot study [14]. This finding calls for validation in larger trials and in different groups of cardiovascular risk patients, especially in patients with impaired fasting glucose or type 2 diabetes.

As insulin resistance is a major factor behind metabolic abnormalities and hemodynamic changes in obese changes, it has been given advice that weight control should be an important part of the reduction in insulin resistance and the correction of these abnormalities. A recent document from European organizations has pointed out the importance of the prevention and treatment of obesity [15]. This is also relevant for prevention of resistant hypertension. Other lifestyle improvements are also of importance to reach this goal, for example, increased physical activity and smoking cessation. Already almost 30 years ago it was shown that smoking is a factor that might increase the degree of dyslipidemia found in most patients with hypertension, especially combined with abdominal obesity [16]. Smoking is also a factor that might aggravate increased activity in the cortisol system, of great importance for metabolic regulation [17]. Besides that, smokers are sometimes not only ignorant of their own lifestyle but also of regular drug intake as prescribed by their physicians. Therefore, smoking cessation has the potential to improve self-respect and increase willingness also to be adherent to the prescribed drug therapy, for example, to control hypertension.

13.6 Diabetes and Resistant Hypertension

There is evidence that diabetes in poor regulation is associated with resistant hypertension. In one study of 10,526 individuals with completed sleep surveys participating in a screening study [18], the authors identified 379 patients with severe hypertension defined as those treated with $\geq$3 antihypertensive medications including a diuretic. In total, 110 of these patients had resistant hypertension despite therapy, while 269 were controlled for severe hypertension. Patients with this condition were more likely to be married, less educated, smoke, self-report unsatisfactory health, and diabetes when compared with patients with controlled hypertension. Multivariate analyses showed that poorly controlled diabetes (glycated hemoglobin more than 7 %) was the factor most strongly associated with resistant hypertension (OR: 3.0; 95 % CI 1.2–7.9). Unsatisfactory health (OR: 1.7; 95 % CI 1.7–2.7) was also associated with resistant hypertension. Poorly controlled diabetes and self-reported unsatisfactory heath showed significant association with this condition. Contrary to expectations, there was no significant association between self-reported snoring and resistant hypertension, when other factors were examined. The documented association between poorly controlled diabetes and resistant hypertension motivates further emphasis on strict control of diabetes in these individuals [18].

13.7 Data from the National Diabetes Register in Sweden

The National Diabetes Register (NDR) was initiated in 1996 as a tool for local quality assurance and feedback in diabetes care. Annual reporting to the NDR is carried out by trained physicians and nurses via the Internet or via clinical records databases, with information collected during patient visits at hospital outpatient clinics and primary health care centers nationwide. All included patients have agreed by informed consent to register before inclusion. Reports concerning blood pressure control and risk of cardiovascular disease in the NDR have been published previously [19, 20].

This observational sub-study of NDR included 6,216 patients with type 2 diabetes on antihypertensive drug treatment, aged 30–80 years, with data available for all analyzed variables between 2005 and 2006, and with at least three drug prescriptions used during this period. In each patient, baseline was defined as occurring after 12 months of continuous use of the prescribed antihypertensive medication. Exclusion criteria were history before baseline of CHD, stroke, heart failure, atrial fibrillation, peripheral vascular disease, amputation, renal failure, gastric/duodenal/peptic ulcer, all forms of cancer, as well as BMI <18 kg/m^2 and serum creatinine >150 μmol/l. The definition of type 2 diabetes was treatment with diet only, oral hypoglycemic agents only, or onset age of diabetes ≥ 40 years and insulin only or combined with oral agents. Only 1 % had onset age <30 years, and 3 % had onset age <40 years. Study information was linked from four national registers in Sweden: the NDR, the Prescribed Drug Register, the Cause of Death Register, and the Hospital Discharge Register at the National Board of Health and Welfare.

All patients on antihypertensive drug treatment were divided into two subgroups, 1,569 patients with resistant hypertension and 4,426 patients without resistant hypertension and with controlled blood pressure <140/90 mmHg. Resistant hypertension was defined as treatment with at least 3 antihypertensive drugs among which one of them was a diuretic, and blood pressure $\geq$140/90 mmHg at baseline. Clinical characteristics included at baseline in 2005–2006: age, gender, diabetes duration, previous hospitalization, type of hypoglycemic treatment, HbA_{1c}, weight, height, smoking, systolic blood pressure, total cholesterol, HDL cholesterol, cumulative microalbuminuria, use of antihypertensive drugs, statins and other lipid-lowering drugs, aspirin use, cardiac glycosides, organic nitrates, and multidose dispensation. BMI (kg/m^2) was calculated as weight/height^2. The Swedish standard for blood pressure recording, used in the NDR, is the mean (mm Hg) of two readings (Korotkoff 1–5) with a cuff of appropriate size, after at least 5 min of rest. A smoker was defined as a patient smoking one or more cigarettes/day, or smoking tobacco using a pipe, or stopped smoking within the past three months. Aspirin treatment was defined as daily oral intake of 75–160 mg acetyl salicylic acid per day. Laboratory analyses of HbA_{1c} and serum lipids were carried out at local laboratories. HbA_{1c} analyses are quality assured nationwide by regular calibration with the HPLC Mono-S method. HbA_{1c}

Table 13.1 Baseline characteristics of two sub-groups, with resistant or controlled hypertension, out of 6,216 treated hypertensive (HT) patients with type 2 diabetes, aged 30–80 years, from the National Diabetes Register (NDR) of Sweden

	Resistant HT	Controlled HT	*P* value
Numbers	1,790	4,426	
Age, years	66.0 ± 8.0	63.1 ± 9.0	<0.001
Diabetes duration, years	8.3 ± 6.7	7.2 ± 6.3	<0.001
Systolic BP, mmHg	153.9 ± 14	127.7 ± 7	<0.001
Diastolic BP, mmHg	81.0 ± 9.8	74.4 ± 7.5	<0.001
HbA_{1c}, %	7.2 ± 1.1	7.0 ± 1.1	<0.001
BMI, kg/m^2	30.8 ± 5.1	30.2 ± 5.2	<0.001
Total cholesterol, mmol/l	4.84 ± 0.9	4.85 ± 0.93	0.6
HDL cholesterol, mmol/l	1.33 ± 0.39	1.34 ± 0.39	0.3
Ratio total:HDL cholesterol	3.87 ± 1.17	3.87 ± 1.27	0.8
Male gender	51.6	54.1	0.08
Smoking	11.7	15.3	<0.001
Albuminuria >20 μg/min	30.1	22.5	<0.001
Previous hospitalization	4.2	4.7	0.4
Hypoglycemic treatment			
Oral agents only	44.2	46.7	0.07
Oral agents and insulin	23.5	16.0	<0.001
Insulin only	11.1	11.7	0.5
ACE inhibitors	31.2	32.4	0.3
ACE inhibitors + diuretics	15.9	4.8	<0.001
ACE inhib + Ca antagonists	0	0.05	0.3
AT2 antagonists	17.9	16.7	0.2
AT2 antagonists + diuretics	32.2	8.8	<0.001
Ca antagonists	61.6	24.4	<0.001
Beta receptor blockers	73.4	39.1	<0.001
Diuretics	57.3	27.4	<0.001
Alpha receptor blockers	3.6	1.1	<0.001
Organic nitrates	3.8	3.6	0.7
Cardiac glycosides	1.3	0.5	<0.001
ASA	46.2	35.3	<0.001

(continued)

Table 13.1 (continued)

	Resistant HT	Controlled HT	*P* value
Statins	51.4	46.3	<0.001
Other lipid-lowering drugs	2.7	2.6	0.8
Estrogen	6.0	5.7	0.7
Multidose dispensation	0.9	0.9	0.9

Mean ± SD and frequencies (%) are given. Crude significance is calculated using Student's *t* test or chi-squared test. Resistant hypertension and controlled hypertension were defined as stated in Methods

values were converted to the DCCT standard values using the formula: HbA_{1c} (DCCT) = 0.923× HbA_{1c} (Mono-S) + 1.345; $R^2 = 0.998$. Albuminuria was defined as cumulative microalbuminuria: urine albumin excretion >20 μg/L.

Statistical methods: Clinical characteristics are presented as means ±1 standard deviation (SD) or frequencies in Table 13.1, with crude significance levels of differences in patients with or without resistant hypertension, when analyzed with use of student's *t* test or X^2 test. All statistical analyses were performed with SAS version 9.3 (SAS Institute, Cary, NC, USA). A p value <0.05 at two-sided test was considered statistically significant in two out of three consecutive tests.

13.8 Results and Interpretation

The patients with diabetes and resistant hypertension were older and showed higher levels of risk factors as compared to controls (Table 13.1). A long-term cardiovascular risk associated with resistant hypertension was suggested by the risk factor cluster and increased drug use associated with resistant hypertension. This is the subject of further follow-up studies now ongoing.

In patients with diabetes, the occurrence of resistant hypertension is thus associated with an increased risk factor burden that may explain any risk increase in cardiovascular events.

13.9 Conclusion

In summary, there is evidence to show that patients with resistant hypertension most often are also characterized by metabolic abnormalities, especially abnormal glucose metabolism or type 2 diabetes, insulin resistance, and dyslipidemia. This is influenced by other contributing factors such as overt abdominal obesity, OSA, hyperaldosteronism, hypercortisolemia, and abnormal autonomic nervous function. Lifestyle improvements, treatment of OSA, and correction of sympathetic over-activation are ways to correct not only resistant hypertension but also the metabolic alterations that are associated with this condition. Further epidemiological studies should aim to describe the prevalence of resistant hypertension in various populations, and in specific risk groups such as patients with type 2 diabetes.

Acknowledgments We thank all participating patients, regional coordinators, nurses, and physicians who have contributed to the NDR study. The NDR is supported by the Swedish Society for Diabetology and the Swedish Diabetes Federation. The Swedish Board of Health and Welfare funds the NDR.
There were no conflicts of interest.

References

1. Isaksson H, Danielsson M, Rosenhamer G, Konarski-Svensson JC, Ostergren J (1991) Characteristics of patients resistant to antihypertensive drug therapy. J Intern Med 229:421–426
2. Isaksson H, Cederholm T, Jansson E, Nygren A, Ostergren J (1993) Therapy-resistant hypertension associated with central obesity, insulin resistance, and large muscle fibre area. Blood Press 2:46–52
3. Isaksson H, Konarski K, Theorell T (1992) The psychological and social condition of hypertensives resistant to pharmacological treatment. Soc Sci Med 35:869–875
4. Isaksson H, Ostergren J (1994) Prognosis in therapy-resistant hypertension. J Intern Med 236:643–649
5. Armario P, Oliveras A, Hernández Del Rey R, Ruilope LM, De La Sierra A (2011) Grupo de Investigadores del Registro de Hipertensión refractaria de la Sociedad Española de Hipertensión/Liga Española para la Lucha contra la Hipertensión Arterial (SEH-LELHA). (Prevalence of target organ damage and metabolic abnormalities in resistant hypertension). Med Clin (Barc) 137:435–439
6. de la Sierra A, Segura J, Banegas JR, Gorostidi M, de la Cruz JJ, Armario P, Oliveras A, Ruilope LM (2011) Clinical features of 8,295 patients with resistant hypertension classified on the basis of ambulatory blood pressure monitoring. Hypertension 57:898–902
7. de la Sierra A, Banegas JR, Oliveras A, Gorostidi M, Segura J, de la Cruz JJ, Armario P, Ruilope LM (2012) Clinical differences between resistant hypertensives and patients treated and controlled with three or less drugs. J Hypertens 30:1211–1216
8. Parati G, Lombardi C, Hedner J, Bonsignore MR, Grote L, Tkacova R, Levy P, Riha R, Bassetti C, Narkiewicz K, Mancia G, McNicholas WT (2012) European Respiratory Society; EU COST ACTION B26 members (2012). Position paper on the management of patients with obstructive sleep apnea and hypertension: joint recommendations by the European Society of Hypertension, by the European Respiratory Society and by the members of European COST (Cooperation in Scientific and Technological research) ACTION B26 on obstructive sleep apnea. J Hypertens 30:633–646
9. Li NF, Yao XG, Zhu J, Yang J, Liu KJ, Wang YC, Wang XL, Zu FY (2010) Higher levels of plasma TNF-alpha and neuropeptide Y in hypertensive patients with obstructive sleep apnea syndrome. Clin Exp Hypertens 32:54–60
10. Viera AJ (2012) Resistant hypertension. J Am Board Fam Med 25:487–495
11. Monticone S, Viola A, Tizzani D, Crudo V, Burrello J, Galmozzi M, Veglio F, Mulatero P (2012) Primary aldosteronism: who should be screened? Horm Metab Res 44:163–169
12. Whaley-Connell A, Johnson MS, Sowers JR (2010) Aldosterone: role in the cardiometabolic syndrome and resistant hypertension. Prog Cardiovasc Dis 52:401–409
13. Boer-Martins L, Figueiredo VN, Demacq C, Martins LC, Consolin-Colombo F, Figueiredo MJ et al (2011) Relationship of autonomic imbalance and circadian disruption with obesity and type 2 diabetes in resistant hypertensive patients. Cardiovasc Diabetol 10:24

14. Mahfoud F, Schlaich M, Kindermann I, Ukena C, Cremers B, Brandt MC et al (2011) Effect of renal sympathetic denervation on glucose metabolism in patients with resistant hypertension: a pilot study. Circulation 123:1940–1946
15. Jordan J, Yumuk V, Schlaich M, Nilsson PM, Zahorska-Markiewicz B, Grassi G et al (2012) Joint statement of the European Association for the study of obesity and the European Society of hypertension: obesity and difficult to treat arterial hypertension. J Hypertens 30:1047–1055
16. Halkin H, Or J, Fuchs Z, Lusky A, Chetrit A, Modan M (1989) Smoking accounts for adverse effect of antihypertensive medications on plasma lipids. A population-based study. Hypertension 14:210–217
17. Pereira CD, Azevedo I, Monteiro R, Martins MJ (2012) 11β-Hydroxysteroid dehydrogenase type 1: relevance of its modulation in the pathophysiology of obesity, the metabolic syndrome and type 2 diabetes mellitus. Diabetes Obes Metab doi:10.1111/j.1463-1326.2012.01582.x (Epub ahead of print)
18. Walia H, Strohl K, Koo B, Seicean A, Seicean S (2012) Are sleep symptoms predictors of resistant hypertension in a population-based sample? Findings from the national health and nutritional examination survey. J Clin Hypertens (Greenwich) 14:530–536
19. Nilsson PM, Cederholm J, Zethelius B, Eliasson B, Eeg-Olofsson K, Gudbjörnsdottir S (2011) Trends in blood pressure control in patients with type 2 diabetes-data from the Swedish National Diabetes Register (NDR). Blood Press 20:348–354
20. Cederholm J, Gudbjörnsdottir S, Eliasson B, Zethelius B, Eeg-Olofsson K, Nilsson PM; on behalf of the NDR (2012). Blood pressure and risk of cardiovascular diseases in type 2 diabetes: further findings from the Swedish National Diabetes Register (NDR-BP II). J Hypertens (Epub ahead of print)

Follow-up of Patients with Resistant Hypertension

14

Manolis S. Kallistratos, Antonios N. Pavlidis
and Athanasios J. Manolis

14.1 Introduction

Resistant hypertension (RH) is defined as failure to reach goal BP in spite of concurrent treatment with maximum tolerated doses of three antihypertensive agents of different classes, including a diuretic [1]. It is of great importance clinicians not to confound RH with uncontrolled hypertension. The latter includes patients with poorly treated BP due to inadequate medical therapy, inappropriate lifestyle habits, or poor adherence to medication; however, a subcategory suffers from true RH [1, 2].

The exact prevalence of RH is difficult to be determined and a forced titration study of a large, diverse hypertensive cohort is necessary in order to be established. In several trials, 20–35 % of participants could not achieve BP control despite receiving more than three antihypertensive medications [3–6].

Although no studies have yet addressed prognosis, it could be assumed that patients with RH are at high cardiovascular risk. Evidence from population studies shows that target organ damage as well as morbidity and mortality is strictly related to the level of BP [6, 7]. Nevertheless, the effects of treatment of RH on morbidity and mortality are still unknown.

M. S. Kallistratos · A. J. Manolis (✉)
Cardiology Department of Asklepeion General Hospital,
Vasileos Pavlou 1 Voula, 16673 Athens, Greece
e-mail: ajmanol@otenet.gr

M. S. Kallistratos
e-mail: Kallistrat1972@gmail.com

A. N. Pavlidis
Cardiology Department, St Thomas' Hospital, Westminster Bridge Road,
London, SE1 7EH, UK
e-mail: antonispav@yahoo.com

G. Mancia (ed.), *Resistant Hypertension*, DOI: 10.1007/978-88-470-5415-8_14,

Table 14.1 Common causes of resistant hypertension

Common conditions	*Exogenous substances*
Older age	Excess alcohol consumption
Obesity	Excess sodium intake
Smoking	Drugs
Diabetes mellitus	
Inadequate treatment	
Pseudo-resistant hypertension	*Secondary hypertension*
Measurement artifact	Renal parenchymal disease
Patient compliance	Renovascular disease
White-coat hypertension	Primary aldosteronism
Pseudohypertension	Obstructive sleep apnea
	Cushing's disease
	Thyroid and parathyroid disease
	Pheochromocytoma

Several trials have demonstrated that achievement of BP goals is still poor despite the use of several protocol-defined treatment regimens. Follow-up of these patients seems to be even more difficult since there are practically no data regarding long-term surveillance of patients with RH. This article provides an overview on the assessment and follow-up of patients with resistant hypertension.

Key elements of monitoring and follow-up, are based on the avoidance of all factors that can increase blood pressure levels (Table 14.1), on prevention, on lifestyle modifications, and of course on knowledge of pharmacological treatment that must be applied in order to maintain blood pressure levels within desired limits.

14.2 Factors that can Increase Blood Pressure Levels

Numerous factors related to the physician or to the patient have been identified as causes of increased blood pressure in patients with RH. Although the term pseudo-resistant hypertension refers to failure to control BP with appropriate antihypertensive treatment in patients who do not truly suffer from RH, those same factors must be avoid in the follow-up of a patient with RH.

Inaccurate BP measurement is the most frequently observed. Common mistakes include as follows:

1. Measure BP before the patient has seated and relaxed for at least 5 min,
2. Failure to support the arm at the level of the heart,

3. Obtain a single instead of at least two readings,
4. Measure BP shortly after the patient has consumed tobacco, and
5. Use of an undersized cuff resulting into falsely high BP readings [8, 9].

Pseudohypertension is a term used to describe high BP readings that do not correlate to interarterial BP measurements and result from the inadequate cuff compression of the heavily calcified arteries, usually in older patients, leading to overestimation of BP [10]. *White-coat hypertension* has also been identified as a cause of pseudo-resistant hypertension and is determined by constant high office BP readings but normal home or ambulatory measurements. This is a very common finding among patients with RH with an incidence that reaches approximately 30 % [11, 12]. While patients with RH due to white-coat hypertension have a better prognosis compared to patients with true hypertension and demonstrate less organ damage, they carry a higher morbidity compared to healthy individuals [13].

14.2.1 Patient Compliance

Poor patient adherence and compliance to antihypertensive treatment is another cause of RH and can be extremely crucial in inadequate BP control. Approximately 40 % of the newly diagnosed hypertensive patients will discontinue their treatment during the first year due to its complexity or the side effects, and only a 40 % of them will continue to be on antihypertensive therapy over the next decade [14–16]. Inappropriate or insufficient patient education regarding the benefits of achieving BP goals, the potential side effects of the prescribed medications, and the high cost of treatment has been highlighted as the most common reasons for self-discontinuation of antihypertensive therapy [17]. Patients must be instructed to bring all their medicines in every visit, giving them the opportunity to review the dose regiment as well as to reconcile medication lists.

14.2.2 Obesity

Obesity has also been linked to RH. Mechanisms of obesity-induced hypertension include increased sympathetic nervous system activity and activation of the renin–angiotensin–aldosterone system (RAAS) [18]. Insulin resistance, hyperinsulinemia, impaired sodium excretion, increased aldosterone sensitivity related to visceral adiposity, and obstructive sleep apnea have all been implicated as potential causes of hypertension in obese subjects [19–21]. It has been shown that as body mass index increases, progressively higher doses of antihypertensive drugs are required in order to achieve optimal BP control [22]. On the other hand, several studies have shown that weight loss is associated with BP reduction in obese hypertensive patients [9]. These reductions are even greater in patients already receiving antihypertensive therapy [23].

14.2.3 Diet

Dietary factors such as increased alcohol and salt consumption contribute to the presence of RH. Modest alcohol consumption, approximately two drinks per day, causes peripheral vasodilation and can reduce BP. However, larger amounts such as three or more drinks per day demonstrate a dose-related effect on BP, both in hypertensive and normotensive persons [24]. In a cross-sectional analysis of Chinese adults consuming more than 30 drinks per week, the risk of hypertension increased from 12 to 14 % [25]. Cessation of heavy alcohol consumption reduced systolic BP by 7.2 mmHg and diastolic BP by 6.6 mmHg, while the prevalence of hypertension declined from 42 to 12 % [26].

The majority of RH patients demonstrate higher salt intake compared to the general population, exceeding the amount of 10 g/day in average [27]. Salt consumption increases BP and blunts the BP lowering effect of most classes of antihypertensive agents [28]. These effects tend to be more pronounced in typical salt-sensitive patients, including the elderly, African-Americans, and particularly patients with chronic kidney disease [29]. It is recommended that dietary sodium in hypertensive patients should be restricted to a maximum of 100 mmol/day (2.4 g sodium or 6 g sodium chloride) and even lower in salt-sensitive patients [30].

14.2.4 Drugs

Several commonly used medications can raise BP and hinder treatment (Table 14.2). Nonnarcotic analgesics, including nonsteroidal anti-inflammatory

Table 14.2 Drugs that can cause resistant hypertension

Nonsteroidal anti-inflammatory drugs	Steroid hormones
Nicotine	Tricyclic antidepressants
Cocaine	Erythropoietin
Caffeine	Phenothiazines
Stimulants	Dietary and herbal supplements
• Methylphenidate	• Ginseng
• Dexmethylphenidate	• Yohimbine
	• Ma huang
• Dextroamphetamine	• Bitter orange
• Amphetamine	
• Methamphetamine	
• Modafinil	
Sympathomimetics	
• Decongestants	
• Anorectics	

agents (NSAIDs), aspirin, and acetaminophen, are probably the most common offending agents in terms of worsening BP control [31]. NSAIDs increase mean arterial pressure by approximately 5 mmHg and may blunt antihypertensive effect of several categories of medications, including diuretics, angiotensin–converting enzyme inhibitors (ACE inhibitors), angiotensin receptor blockers [ARBs], and b-blockers [32–34]. The effect of NSAIDs on BP is more pronounced in patients with impaired renal function [1]. Decongestant agents such as phenylephrine and pseudoephedrine and stimulant agents used for weight loss have also been implicated in increasing BP. Contraceptives, cyclosporine, erythropoietin, and cortisone raise BP via fluid retention, particularly in patients with increased mineralocorticoid activity [1].

14.3 Lifestyle Changes

Lifestyle changes, including weight reduction, regular exercise, and moderate alcohol and salt consumption, should be encouraged where suitable. Weight loss can reduce BP and increase functional capacity [35, 36]. A 10-kg weight loss is associated with an average reduction of 6 mmHg in systolic and 4.6 mmHg in diastolic BP [36]. Physical activity can decrease systolic and diastolic BP by 7 and 5 mmHg, respectively, in patients with RH [37]. A modest alcohol intake can also decrease BP levels.

Habitual alcohol intake is associated with raised morning BP readings, increased heart rate throughout the day, and increased sympathetic activity during sleep. These findings can partially explain the link of heavy alcohol consumption to an increased risk of cardiovascular diseases [38]. Daily alcohol consumption should be restricted to two units per day for men and one unit per day for women or patients with low body mass index [39].

Dietary salt restriction decreases systolic and diastolic BP levels in hypertensive patients by 5–10 mmHg and 2–6 mmHg, respectively [40, 41]. Ideally, sodium consumption should be restricted to less than 100 mEq/day for all patients with RH [1].

14.4 Prevention

Different risk factors frequently appear in the same individual. Only a small fraction of patients suffers from hypertension without presenting other risk factors (24 %) [42]. Patients with RH are assumed to be high-risk patients. Evidence from population studies shows that target organ damage as well as morbidity and mortality is strictly related to the level of BP [6, 7]. Several studies like NHANES study [43] and the SPANISH study [44] showed that patients with resistant hypertension had higher rates of renal dysfunction, albuminuria as well as increased cardiovascular morbidity and mortality. Although, the effects of treatment of RH on morbidity and mortality are still unknown, physicians should focus on prevention and reduction in risk factors as well as revealing target organ damage since the majority of the patients present overlapping risk factors and associated co morbidities. Risk estimation is facilitated using risk charts such as SCORE that estimates the 10-year risk of a first fatal atherosclerotic event, whether heart attack, stroke, aneurysm of the aorta, or other [9]. Thus, patients should be classified in relation of the total cardiovascular risk resulting from the coexistence of different risk factors, organ damage, and disease [9].

14.5 Secondary Hypertension

Usually secondary causes of hypertension (SH) are considered and rule out during the initial evaluation of a patient with newly diagnosed hypertension. However, patients with RH represent a population with increased rates of SH especially in the elderly. Specific biochemical disturbances, such as hypokalemia and metabolic alkalosis, or physical signs such as central obesity, purple striae, and abdominal bruits may suggest a secondary cause of hypertension [45]. A long list of secondary causes of hypertension exists in the literature, although some of them are rarely encountered in every day clinical practice. Renal parenchymal disease is the most common cause of secondary hypertension (SH) and can complicate treatment and prognosis. In the ALLHAT trial, serum creatinine levels above 1.5 mg/dL were the strongest predictor of failure to achieve goal BP [46]. RH results from activation of the sympathetic nervous system and the RAAS, sodium retention, and intravascular volume expansion [47].

Renovascular hypertension is a relatively common cause of SH. Its prevalence is estimated between 1 and 5 % of all hypertensive patients in the general population and can reach up to 30 % in a highly selected referral population. Renovascular hypertension may be caused by a heterogeneous group of disorders, but the most common are fibromuscular dysplasia and atherosclerotic renovascular disease [48–51].

Primary aldosteronism is caused by autonomous production of aldosterone by the adrenal cortex. Its incidence varies between 1 and 11 % in patients with hypertension [52]. In 65–90 % of the cases primary aldosteronism occurs in the setting of aldosterone secreting adrenal adenomas. The aldosteronoma is solitary in 65–70 % of the cases, multiple adenomas are present in 13 % and microadenoma exists in 6 % of the patients [53, 54]. Primary aldosteronism is characterized by moderate to severe hypertension without the presence of peripheral edema. The diagnosis is based on the typical biochemical finding of hypokalemia, hypernatremia, magnesium depletion, elevated bicarbonate levels, low plasma pH, and elevated aldosterone levels in the serum and urine [45].

Obstructive sleep apnea (OSA) represents an independent risk factor for the development of hypertension [55]. In patients with RH, a significant percentage suffers from OSA [56]. Repeated episodes of sleep apnea result in periodic hypoxia and increased sympathetic activity, heart rate ,and blood pressure. Those factors contribute to the development or progression of hypertension [56]. Polysonography represents the gold standard for the diagnosis of OSA; however, questionnaires like the Epworth Sleepiness Scale or the sleep apnea clinical score could be a cost-effective alternative for screening those patients [57–59].

Early recognition and treatment of the various causes of SH can reduce BP levels and in some cases abolish hypertension [1]. In patients with RH and sleep apnea syndrome, the use of nasal C-PAP for 2 months is associated with a reduction in nighttime and daytime ambulatory systolic BP (14.4 and 9.3 mmHg, respectively) and a 7.8 mmHg reduction in nighttime diastolic BP [60].

Patients with renal artery stenosis may benefit from angioplasty, although the results of endovascular revascularization are controversial. The relative benefit of intensive medical therapy compared to interventional treatment has not been clearly established [61]. Revascularization may fail to cure hypertension when stenoses are long-standing [62]. Moreover, in the absence of complete vascular occlusion, the correlation between the amount of stenosis and glomerular filtration rate has been inconsistent [63]. When RH is caused by primary aldosteronism, pheochromocytoma, or Cushing's disease, treatment should be guided accordingly.

14.6 Pharmacological Treatment

The knowledge of pharmacological treatment that must be applied in patients with RH is imperative in order to maintain blood pressure levels within desired limits.

To improve patient compliance to antihypertensive treatment, physicians should prescribe simple, fewer, and more effective regiments such as long-acting agents and fixed-dose combinations. Fixed-dose combinations not only improve patient compliance but also decrease the incidence of drug-related side effects. They can also provide more reliable BP control due to the synergic effect of the different classes of agents contained [64]. When combining antihypertensive drugs, the complimentary mechanisms of action should always be considered. The optimal regimen will likely include agents from several classes that target different pathophysiological pathways.

Patients with RH should strictly avoid medications that may reduce the action of antihypertensive drugs, such as NSAIDs. When the use of these drugs is inevitable, substances with minimal interference are recommended (e.g., acetaminophen) [65]. Nevertheless, BP should be monitored closely irrespectively of the final choice. The scheduled time of drug administration can also affect BP control. Administration of one antihypertensive at night may normalize BP in 22–37 % of the patients. This effect is even more pronounced in nondippers [66, 67].

Volume overload is the most frequent cause of RH. Optimizing or changing diuretic therapy can increase the percentage of patients who achieves target BP [68]. In patients with RH, unless contraindicated, an appropriate dose of a diuretic should always be included. Several studies have shown that low-dose chlorthalidone (12.5–25 mg/day) is more effective than hydrochlorothiazide [69, 70]. Additionally, in a small study of patients with RH, switching from the same dose of hydrochlorothiazide to chlorthalidone resulted in an additional 8 mmHg drop in systolic BP and increased the number of patients that achieved target BP levels [71]. In patients with renal impairment and glomerular filtration rate (GFR), < 40 ml/min/1.73 m^2 administration of a loop diuretic, such as furosemide, bumetanide, and torasemide, should be considered taking into account the short durations of action of the first two [3–6 h].

Aldosterone is also part of the RAAS, and the use of an aldosterone antagonist (spironolactone or eplerenone) can be helpful in controlling BP in patients with RH [72]. The magnitude of BP decrease is similar in patients with RH and primary hyperaldosteronism [73, 74]. Spironolactone is usually initiated at 12.5–25 mg/day and can be titrated up to 50 mg/day at 4–6-week intervals. Doses higher than 50 mg/day have not been studied in RH, but have shown benefits in patients with true hyperaldosteronism [72]. Spironolactone is a low-cost aldosterone antagonist that can cause tender gynecomastia [73]. This is a dose-related effect and usually occurs in doses higher than 50 mg/day. Gynecomastia is much less frequent with eplerenone; however, no data exist regarding its use in RH patients. As with spironolactone, the antihypertensive response to eplerenone does not appear to be related to underlying plasma aldosterone or rennin levels [74, 75].

Amiloride is a potassium-sparing diuretic associated with satisfactory BP lowering results in patients with RH [76]. It acts by antagonizing the epithelial sodium channel in the distal collecting duct of the kidney and thereby functions as an indirect aldosterone antagonist. When potassium-sparing diuretics are prescribed in addition to an ACE inhibitor or an ARB, potassium levels should be closely monitored, especially in patients with impaired renal function. Patients should also be advised against consumption of foods and supplements that are rich in potassium.

Alpha blockers (hydralazine or minoxidil) and combined alpha–beta receptor blockers (e.g., labetalol) can provide additional antihypertensive effect when added to existing regimens in patients with RH [9]. Centrally acting alpha-agonists (methyldopa and clonidine) can also be effective; however, tolerability issues exist and frequent dosing is a disadvantage. Minoxidil can cause hypertrichosis as well as rush, swelling of the mouth, and light-headedness. With minoxidil, concomitant use of a b-blocker and a loop diuretic is usually required due to reflex tachycardia and fluid retention.

For patients with true RH, there are data to support the addition of a calcium channel blocker (CCB) to a regimen that includes a RAAS blocker and a diuretic. This results in additive BP reduction with low side-effect incidence [77, 78]. Combining an ACE inhibitor with an ARB seems to be less effective in terms of BP reduction compared to a combination of CCB and ARB [79]. In addition, the combination of ACE inhibitor and ARB does not further reduce cardiovascular or renal events compared to monotherapy with wither agent and may confer an increased risk of side effects [80, 81].

14.6.1 Novel Antihypertensives

Endothelin receptor antagonists consist a new family of antihypertensive medications. Darusentan is a selective antagonist of type A endothelin receptors that causes vasoconstriction and proliferation of vascular smooth muscles [82]. This agent demonstrated a dose dependent decrease in BP, while the greatest reductions (11.5 and 6.3 mmHg for systolic and diastolic BP, respectively) were observed after 10 weeks of high-dose treatment [83]. Omapatrilat is a neutral endopeptidase inhibitor that showed favorable antihypertensive effects in the OCTAVE trial [84]. Moreover, vaccines targeting angiotensin I and II are also being developed and tested with promising initial results [85].

14.6.2 Device Therapy for Patients with Resistant Hypertension

The Rheos system is a pacemaker-like device intended for surgical implantation in the carotid with the aim of activating the baroreflex and reducing blood pressure. Recent studies in both normotensive and hypertensive canine models have demonstrated sustained and clinically relevant reductions in arterial pressure and sympathetic activity with prolonged baroreflex activation [86, 87]. However, this novel approach is under evaluation, and more epidemiological studies with larger samples are expected.

14.6.3 Renal Denervation

Before antihypertensive drugs became generally available, nonselective surgical sympathectomy was effectively used as a treatment of severe hypertension [86]. Renal sympathetic efferent and afferent nerves are crucial for the initiation and maintenance of systemic hypertension and lie within and immediately adjacent to the wall of the renal artery [88]. Recently developed endovascular catheter technology enables selective denervation of the human kidney, with radiofrequency energy with promising results. Catheter-based renal denervation in the multicentre Simplicity HTN-1 study, decrease mean blood pressure by 33/15 mmHg at 24 months without evidence of vascular, or renal abnormalities in patients with persistently elevated blood pressure despite treatment with an average of five medications, without evidence of vascular or renal abnormalities [89]. HTN-2 study showed similar results [90]. Proposed steps for follow-up of a patient with resistant hypertension are shown in Table 14.3.

Table 14.3 Proposed steps for patients with resistant hypertension (RH)

• Obtain a detailed past medical history and perform all necessary clinical investigations to rule out secondary causes of RH (if suspected)
• Confirm compliance and exclude pseudo-resistant hypertension or drug-induced RH
• Perform proper office BP measurements and consider ambulatory BP to rule out white-coat hypertension or inappropriate home BP measurements
• Discontinue or minimize interfering medications
• Identify possible contributing lifestyle-related causes
• Identify possible presence of target organ damage
• Proceed accordingly to lifestyle modifications
• Classify patients in relation of the total cardiovascular risk
• Modify treatment according to patient characteristics using optimal doses of appropriate medications
• Consult a hypertension specialist when BP is not controlled adequately

14.7 Conclusions

RH is a challenging diagnosis which physicians common encounter in clinical practice. Follow-up seems to be equally difficult due to the complexity of those patients. Patient characteristics and comorbidities usually determine the appropriate combination of antihypertensive agents in order to achieve target BP levels. Treatment should be decided on an individual basis in order to maintain an adequate BP control and minimize complications and adverse effects.

References

1. Calhoun DA, Jones D, Textor S et al (2008) Resistant hypertension: diagnosis, evaluation, and treatment, a scientific statement from the American heart association professional education committee of the council for high blood pressure research. Hypertension 51:1403–1419
2. Epstein M (2007) Resistant hypertension: prevalence and evolving concepts. J Clin Hypertens (Greenwich) 9:2–6
3. ALLHAT officers and coordinators for the ALLHAT collaborative research group (2002) The antihypertensive and lipid-lowering treatment to prevent heart attack trial. Major outcomes in high-risk hypertensive patients randomized to angiotensin-converting enzyme inhibitor or calcium channel blocker versus diuretic: the anti-hypertensive and lipid-lowering treatment to prevent heart attack trial (ALLHAT). JAMA 288:2981–2997
4. Dahlof B, Devereux RB, Kjeldsen SE et al (2002) Cardiovascular morbidity and mortality in the Losartan Intervention For Endpoint reduction in hypertension study (LIFE): a randomised trial against atenolol. Lancet 359:995–1003
5. Pepine CJ, Handberg EM, Cooper-DeHoff RM et al (2003) A calcium antagonist versus a non-calcium antagonist hypertension treatment strategy for patients with coronary artery disease.

The International Verapamil-Trandolapril Study (INVEST): a randomized controlled trial. JAMA 290:2805–2816
6. Lewington S, Clarke R, Qizilbash N et al (2002) Age-specific prevalence of usual blood pressure to vascular mortality: a meta-analysis of individual data for one million adults in 61 prospective studies. Lancet 360:1903–1913
7. Chobanian AV, Bakris GL, Black HR et al (2003) Seventh report of the joint national committee on prevention, detection, evaluation, and treatment of high blood pressure. Hypertension 42:1206–1252
8. Pickering TG, Hall JE, Appel LJ et al (2005) Recommendations for blood pressure measurement in humans and experimental animals: part 1: blood pressure measurement in humans: a statement for professionals from the subcommittee of professional and public education of the American heart association council on high blood pressure research. Circulation 111:697–716
9. Mancia G, De Backer G, Dominiczak A et al (2007) Guidelines for the management of arterial hypertension: the task force for the management of arterial hypertension of the European society of hypertension (ESH) and of the European society of cardiology (ESC). Eur Heart J 28(12):1462–1536
10. Cheng TO (1998) Osler maneuver to detect pseudo hypertension. JAMA 282:943
11. Redon J, Campos C, Narciso ML et al (1998) Prognostic value of ambulatory blood pressure monitoring in refractory hypertension: a prospective study. Hypertension 31:712–718
12. Brown MA, Buddle ML, Martin A (2001) Is resistant hypertension really resistant? Am J Hypertens 14:1263–1269
13. Pierdomenico SD, Lapenna D, Bucci A et al (2005) Cardiovascular outcome in treated hypertensive patients with responder, masked, false resistant and true resistant hypertension. Am J Hypertens 18:1422–1428
14. Mazzaglia G, Mantovani LG, Sturkenboom MC et al (2005) Patterns of persistence with antihypertensive medications in newly diagnosed hypertensive patients in Italy: a retrospective cohort study in primary care. J Hypertens 23:2093–2100
15. Caro JJ, Salas M, Speckman JL, Raggio G, Jackson JD (1999) Persistence with treatment for hypertension in actual practice. CMAJ 160:31–37
16. Van Wijk BL, Klungel OH, Heerdink ER, de Boer A (2005) Rate and determinants of 10 year persistence with antihypertensive drugs. J Hypertens 23:2101–2107
17. Takiya LN, Peterson AM, Finley RS (2004) Meta-analysis of interventions for medication adherence to antihypertensives. Ann Pharmacother 38:1617–1624
18. Hall JE (2003) The kidney, hypertension, and obesity. Hypertension 41:625–633
19. Sarafidis PA (2008) Obesity, insulin resistance and kidney disease risk: insights into the relationship. Curr Opin Nephrol Hypertens 17:450–456
20. Morris MJ (2008) Cardiovascular and metabolic effects of obesity. Clin Exp Pharmacol Physiol 35:416–419
21. Wong C, Marwick TH (2007) Obesity cardiomyopathy: pathogenesis and pathophysiology. Nat Clin Pract Cardiovasc Med 4:436–443
22. Mertens LI, Van Gaal LF (2000) Overweight, obesity, and blood pressure: the effects of modest weight reduction, 8(3):270–278
23. Aucott L, Poobalan A, Smith WC et al (2005) Effects of weight loss in overweight/obese individuals and long-term hypertension outcomes: a systematic review. Hypertension 45:1035–1041
24. Chobanian AV, Bakris GL, Black HR et al (2003) Seventh report of the joint national committee on prevention, detection, evaluation, and treatment of high blood pressure. Hypertension 42:1206–1252
25. Wildman RP, Gu D, Muntner P et al (2005) Alcohol intake and hypertension subtypes in Chinese men. J Hypertens 23:737–743

26. Aguilera MT, de la Sierra A, Coca A et al (1999) Effect of alcohol abstinence on blood pressure: assessment by 24 h ambulatory blood pressure monitoring. Hypertension 33:653–657
27. Nishizaka MK, Pratt-Ubunama M, Zaman MA et al (2005) Validity of plasma aldosterone-to-renin activity ratio in African American and white subjects with resistant hypertension. Am J Hypertens 18:805–812
28. He FJ, MacGregor GA (2004) Effect of longer-term modest salt reduction on blood pressure. Cochrane Database Syst Rev 3:CD004937
29. Boudville N, Ward S, Benaroia M, House AA (2005) Increased sodium intake correlates with greater use of antihypertensive agents by subjects with chronic kidney disease. Am J Hypertens 18:1300–1305
30. Chobanian AV, Bakris GL, Black HR et al (2003) Seventh report of the joint national committee on prevention, detection, evaluation, and treatment of high blood pressure. Hypertension 42:1206–1252
31. Forman JP, Stampfer MJ, Curhan GC (2005) Non-narcotic analgesic dose and risk of incident hypertension in US women. Hypertension 46:500–507
32. Johnson AG, Nguyen TV, Day RO (1994) Do nonsteroidal anti-inflammatory drugs affect blood pressure? a meta-analysis. Ann Intern Med 121:289–300
33. Radack KL, Deck CC, Bloomfield SS (1987) Ibuprofen interferes with the efficacy of antihypertensive drugs, a randomized, double-blind, placebo-controlled trial of ibuprofen compared with acetaminophen. Ann Intern Med 107:628–635
34. Conlin PR, Moore TJ, Swartz SL et al (2000) Effect of indomethacin on blood pressure lowering by captopril and losartan in hypertensive patients. Hypertension 36:461–465
35. Wessel TR, Arant CB, Olson MB et al (2004) Relationship of physical fitness vs body mass index with coronary artery disease and cardiovascular events in women. JAMA 292:1179–1187
36. Aucott L, Poobalan A, Smith WC et al (2005) Effects of weight loss in overweight/obese individuals and long-term hypertension outcomes: a systematic review. Hypertension 45:1035–1041
37. Kokkinos PF, Narayan P, Colleran JA et al (1995) Effects of regular exercise on blood pressure and left ventricular hypertrophy in African-American men with severe hypertension. N Engl J Med 333:1462–1467
38. Ohira T, Tanigawa T, Tabata M et al (2009) Effects of habitual alcohol intake on ambulatory blood pressure, heart rate, and its variability among Japanese men. Hypertension 53:13–19
39. Chobanian AV, Bakris GL, Black HR et al (2003) National heart, lung, and blood institute joint national committee on prevention, detection, evaluation, and treatment of high blood pressure; national high blood pressure education program coordinating committee, the seventh report of the joint national committee on prevention, detection, evaluation, and treatment of high blood pressure: the JNC 7 report. JAMA 289:2560–2572
40. Neter JE, Stam BE, Kok FJ, Grobbee DE, Geleijnse JM (2003) Influence of weight reduction on blood pressure: a meta-analysis of randomized controlled trials. Hypertension 42:878–884
41. He FJ, Markandu ND, MacGregor GA (2005) Modest salt reduction lowers blood pressure in isolated systolic hypertension and combined hypertension. Hypertension 46:66–70
42. Wong DN, Lopez VA, L'Italien G, Chen R, Kline SE, Franklin SS (2007) Inadequate control of hypertension in US adults with cardiovascular disease comorbidities in 2003–2004. Arch Intern Med 167(22):2431–2436
43. Persell SD (2011) Prevalence of resistant hypertension in the United States, 2003–2008. Hypertens Jun 57(6):1076–1080
44. De la Sierra A, Segura J, Banegas JR, et al (2011) Clinical features of 8,295 patients with resistant hypertension classified on the basis of ambulatory blood pressure monitoring. Hypertension 57:898e902
45. Kallistratos MS, Giannakopoulos A, German V, Manolis AJ (2010) Diagnostic modalities of most common forms of secondary hypertension. Hellenic J Cardiol 51:518–529

46. Cushman WC, Ford CE, Cutler JA et al (2002) Success and predictors of blood pressure control in diverse North American settings: the antihypertensive and lipid-lowering treatment to prevent heart attack trial (ALLHAT). J Clin Hypertens (Greenwich) 4:393–404
47. Campese VM, Mitra N, Sandee D (2006) Hypertension in renal parenchymal disease: why is it so resistant to treatment? Kidney Int 69:967–973
48. Greco BA, Breyer JA (1997) Atherosclerotic ischemic renal disease. Am J Kid Dis 29:167–187
49. Uzu T, Inoue T, Fujii T et al (1997) Prevalence and predictors of renal artery stenosis in patients with myocardial infarction. Am J Kidney Dis 29:733–738
50. Wilms G, Marchal G, Peene P, Baert AL (1990) The angiographic incidence of renal artery stenosis in the arteriosclerotic population. Eur J Radiol 10:195–197
51. Hansen KJ, Edwards MS, Craven TE et al (2002) Prevalence of renovascular disease in the elderly: a population-based study. J Vasc Surg 36:443–451
52. Rossi GP, Bernini G, Caliumi C et al (2006) PAPY Study investigators, a prospective study of the prevalence of primary aldosteronism in 1,125 hypertensive patients. J Am Coll Cardiol 48:2293–2300
53. Leung AM, Sasano H, Nishikwa T et al (2008) Multiple unilateral adrenal adenomas in a patient with primary hyperaldosteronism. Endocr Pract 14:76–79
54. Pimenta E, Calhoun DA (2007) Resistant hypertension and aldosteronism. Curr Hypertens Rep 9:353–359
55. Peppard PE, Young T, Palta M, Skatrud J (2000) Prospective study of the association between sleep-disordered breathing and hypertension. N Engl J Med 342:1378–1384
56. Logan AG, Perlikowski SM, Mente A (2001) High prevalence of obstructive sleep apnea in drug resistant hypertension. J Hypertension 19:2271–2277
57. Narkiewicz K, van de Borne PJH, Pesek CA, Dyken ME, Montano N, Somers VK (1999) Selective potentiation of peripheral chemoreflex sensitivity in obstructive sleep apnea. Circulation 99:1183–1189
58. Mulgrew AT, Fox N, Ayas NT, Ryan CF (2007) Diagnosis and initial management of obstructive sleep apnea without polysomnography. Ann Intern Med 146:157–166
59. Skomro RP, Gjevre J, Reid J et al (2010) Outcomes of home-based diagnosis and treatment of obstructive sleep apnea. Chest 138(2):257–263
60. Logan AG, Tkacova R, Perlikowski SM et al (2003) Refractory hypertension and sleep apnea: effect of CPAP on blood pressure and baroreflex. Eur Respir J 21:241–247
61. Textor SC (2002) Progressive hypertension in a patient with "incidental" renal artery stenosis. Hypertension 40:595–600
62. O'Donovan RM, Gutierrez OH, Izzo JL Jr (1992) Preservation of renal function by percutaneous renal angioplasty in high-risk elderly patients: short-term outcome. Nephron 60:187–192
63. Suresh M, Laboi P, Mamtora H, Kalra PA (2000) Relationship of renal dysfunction to proximal arterial disease severity in atherosclerotic renovascular disease. Nephrol Dial Transplant 15:631–636
64. Gupta AK, Arshad S, Poulter NR (2010) Compliance, safety, and effectiveness of fixed-dose combinations of antihypertensive agents: a meta-analysis. Hypertension 55:399–407
65. Radack KL, Deck CC, Bloomfield SS (1987) Ibuprofen interferes with the efficacy of antihypertensive drugs, a randomized, double-blind, placebo-controlled trial of ibuprofen compared with acetaminophen. Ann Intern Med 107:628–635
66. Calvo C, Hermida RC, Ayala DE et al (2006) Effects of time-dependent administration of antihypertensive treatment in patients with resistant hypertension. Med Clin (Barc) 126:364–372
67. Hermida RC, Ayala DE, Fernández JR, Calvo C (2008) Chronotherapy improves blood pressure control and reverts the nondipper pattern in patients with resistant hypertension. Hypertension 51:69–76

68. Graves JW, Bloomfield RL, Buckalew VM Jr (1989) Plasma volume in resistant hypertension: guide to pathophysiology and therapy. Am J Med Sci 298:361–365
69. Khosla N, Chua DY, Elliott WJ et al (2005) Are chlorthalidone and hydrochlorothiazide equivalent blood-pressure-lowering medications? J Clin Hypertens 7:354–356
70. Ernst ME, Goerdt CJ, Carter BL et al (2006) Comparative antihypertensive effects of hydrochlorothiazide and chlorthalidone on ambulatory and office blood pressure. Hypertension 47:352–358
71. Khosla N, Chua DY, Elliott WJ, Bakris GL (2005) Are chlorthalidone and hydrochlorothiazide equivalent blood-pressure-lowering medications? J Clin Hypertens (Greenwich) 7:354–356
72. Nishizaka MK, Calhoun DA (2005) The role of aldosterone antagonists in the management of resistant hypertension. Curr Hypertens Rep 7:343–347
73. Nishizaka MK, Zaman MA, Calhoun DA (2003) Efficacy of low-dose Spironolactone in subjects with resistant hypertension. Am J Hypertens 16:925–930
74. Chapman N, Dobson J, Wilson S et al (2007) Effect of spironolactone on blood pressure in subjects with resistant hypertension. Hypertension 49:839–845
75. Krum H, Nolly H, Workman D et al (2007) Efficacy of eplerenone added to renin-angiotensin blockade in hypertensive patients. Hypertension 2002(40):117–123
76. Eide IK, Torjesen PA, Drolsum A, Babovic A, Lilledahl NP (2004) Low-renin status in therapy-resistant hypertension: a clue to efficient treatment. J Hypertens 22:2217–2226
77. Saseen JJ, Carter BL, Brown TE et al (1996) Comparison of nifedipine alone and with diltiazem or verapamil in hypertension. Hypertension 28:109–114
78. Gashti CN, Bakris GL (2004) The role of calcium antagonists in chronic kidney disease. Curr Opin Nephrol Hypertens 13:155–161
79. Stergiou GS, Makris T, Papavasiliou M et al (2005) Comparison of antihypertensive effects of an angiotensin-converting enzyme inhibitor, a calcium antagonist and a diuretic in patients with hypertension not controlled by angiotensin receptor blocker monotherapy. J Hypertens 23:883–889
80. Yusuf S, Teo KK, Pogue J et al (2008) Telmisartan, ramipril, or both in patients at high risk for vascular events. N Engl J Med 358:1547–1559
81. Mann JF, Schmieder R, McQueen M et al (2008) Renal outcomes with telmisartan, ramipril, or both in people at high vascular risk: results from a multicenter, randomised, double-blind, controlled trial. Lancet 372:547–553
82. Black HR, Bakris GL, Weber MA et al (2007) Efficacy and safety of darusentan in patients with resistant hypertension: results from a randomized, double-blind, placebo-controlled dose-ranging study. J Clin Hypertens (Greenwich) 9:760–769
83. Kostis JB, Packer M, Black HR et al (2004) Omapatrilat and enalapril in patients with hypertension: the Omapatrilat cardiovascular treatment vs, Enalapril (OCTAVE) trial. Am J Hypertens 17:103–111
84. Brown MJ, Coltart J, Gunewardena K et al (2004) Randomized double-blind placebo-controlled study of an angiotensin immunotherapeutic vaccine (PMD3117) in hypertensive subjects. Clin Sci (Lond) 107:167–173
85. Ambühl PM, Tissot AC, Fulurija A et al (2007) A vaccine for hypertension based on virus-like particles: preclinical efficacy and phase I safety and immunogenicity. J Hypertens 25:63–72
86. Heusser Karsten, Tank Jens, Engeli Stefan (2010) Carotid baroreceptor stimulation, sympathetic activity, baroreflex function, and blood pressure in hypertensive patients. Hypertension 55:619–626
87. Scheffers IJ, Kroon AA, Schmidli J et al (2010) Novel baroreflex activation therapy in resistant hypertension results of a European multi-center feasibility study. JACC 56(15):1254–1258
88. Campese VM, Kogosov E (1995) Renal afferent denervation prevents hypertension in rats with chronic renal failure part 2, Hypertension 25(4):878–882

89. Krum H, Schlaich M, Whitbourn R et al (2009) Catheter-based renal sympathetic denervation for resistant hypertension: a multicentre safety and proof-of-principle cohort study. Lancet 373(9671):1275–1281
90. Symplicity HTN-2 Investigators (2010) Renal sympathetic denervation in patients with treatment-resistant hypertension (The symplicity HTN-2 Trial): a randomised controlled trial. Lancet 376(9756):1903–9

Resistant Hypertension: Cost-Benefit Considerations

15

Miguel Camafort, Heitor Moreno and Antonio Coca

15.1 Introduction

Health costs are a concern worldwide, and demands for their containment are being made in many countries. There are various approaches to the evaluation of costs and benefits, including cost-effectiveness analysis, cost-utility analysis, which takes into account both the length and the quality of life, and cost-benefit analysis in which both the costs and the outcome (benefit) are measured in monetary terms. While this means that it is possible to see whether a treatment is worthwhile, it is not possible to ascribe a money value to the prolongation and improvement in life. Therefore, cost-effectiveness and, to some extent, cost-benefit analyses are the most frequently employed methods for the evaluation of costs and benefits in the treatment for hypertension.

Hypertension is a common disorder affecting 18 % of adults. Data from trials, such as the STOP [1], SHEP [2], and EWHE [3] trials, and other large clinical trials show that lowering blood pressure (BP) levels significantly reduces the incidence of stroke and myocardial infarction and improves the prognosis of hypertensive patients. Data from the 40-year (1950–1990) Framingham study [4]

M. Camafort · A. Coca (✉)
Hypertension and Vascular Risk Unit, Department of Internal Medicine. Institute of Medicine and Dermatology. Hospital Clínic (IDIBAPS), University of Barcelona, Villarroel 170, Barcelona, 08036 Sao Paulo, Spain
e-mail: acoca@clinic.ub.es

M. Camafort
e-mail: camafort@clinic.ub.es

H. Moreno
Department of Internal Medicine, Faculdade de Ciências Médicas da Universidade Estadual de Campinas—UNICAMP, Campinas 13083-970, Brazil
e-mail: hmoreno@uol.com.br

G. Mancia (ed.), *Resistant Hypertension*, DOI: 10.1007/978-88-470-5415-8_15,

suggest that treatment for sustained hypertension may reduce 10-year all-cause mortality by 41–31 %, with a 10-year risk ratio in treated versus untreated hypertensive subjects of 0.69 (95 % CI 0.53–0.89). An additional approach to the assessment of treatment benefit is the use of intermediate end points such as subclinical organ damage in hypertension. The evidence from studies using such end points may have not the same weight as that based on "hard" end points (fatal and non-fatal myocardial infarction, or fatal and non-fatal stroke, cardiovascular mortality and all-cause mortality). However, a large body of evidence demonstrates that various measures of subclinical organ damage, such as changes in proteinuria and echocardiographic or electrocardiographic left ventricular hypertrophy, have a strong predictive value for subsequent fatal and non-fatal events [5].

Cost-effectiveness analysis can facilitate effective and efficient management of finite healthcare resources in the large population of hypertensive patients, maximizing the effects for a given budget. Early intervention studies clearly demonstrate the benefits of using drug therapy to treat malignant and severe hypertension. Subsequent trials have shown similar results for grade I and II hypertension, although there has been debate on the value or risk and on the cost issues of using the newer classes of antihypertensive drugs [6]. Comparative randomized trials show that, for similar BP reductions, differences in the incidence of cardiovascular morbidity and mortality between different drug classes are small, strengthening the conclusion that their benefit largely depends on BP lowering per se. Due to the failure of several comparative trials to lower BP to the same extent in the two active treatment arms, ESH guideline recommendations have been based on meta-regression analysis in which differences in BP obtained are taken into account [7]. In fact, an overview of all trial evidence suggests that the major classes of antihypertensive drugs are largely equivalent in efficacy and safety. On the other hand, lifestyle measures that should be considered in all patients include reducing salt intake, losing weight in overweight patients, moderation of alcohol consumption, increased physical activity, and an increase in fruit and vegetable intake and a decrease in saturated and total fat intake [8]. However, the evidence that lifestyle changes reduce long-term morbidity and mortality in patients with hypertension is not robust, and long-term compliance in making these changes is low. The cost of drug treatment of hypertension is often contrasted with lifestyle measures, which are considered cost-free. However, real implementation, and therefore effectiveness, of lifestyle changes requires behavioral support, counseling, and reinforcement, which may have a substantial cost.

In addition to obtaining BP levels below the target and reducing mortality and morbidity, treatment should protect against subclinical organ damage, especially the progression of microalbuminuria to overt proteinuria and the development of left ventricular hypertrophy, which both have a strong predictive value for subsequent fatal and non-fatal events. Likewise, as there is evidence of the benefit of treatment over a longer timescale in diabetes, metabolic disorders, and end-stage renal disease [9, 10], antihypertensive treatment should also reduce the impact of these conditions. However, very few clinical studies have assessed these factors.

According to the AHA guidelines on resistant hypertension [11], 24-h ambulatory BP monitoring (ABPM) is the only valid method of differentiating "isolated office-resistant hypertension" from "true resistant hypertension" in patients taking at least three antihypertensive drugs at full doses, including a diuretic. ABPM has the added advantage of providing greater prognostic value than office BP measurements in the evaluation of subjects with resistant hypertension [12]. Therefore, ABPM is essential to improve the cost-effectiveness of the screening, diagnosis, and, indirectly, the treatment for resistant hypertension.

15.2 Cost-Effectiveness of Non-Pharmacological Treatment in Resistant Hypertensive Patients

Obesity is often associated with hypertension, and more than 80 % of patients seen in reference centers have overweight or obesity, particularly those with more severe forms of hypertension. Obesity is associated with a need for an increased number and dose of antihypertensive medications and a greater likelihood of never achieving BP control [13, 14]. As a consequence, obesity is a common feature of patients with resistant hypertension [15]. Obstructive sleep apnea, which is frequently associated with obesity, appears to be the most common condition associated with resistant hypertension [16]. However, randomized evaluations of continuous positive airway pressure (CPAP) indicate an overall modest effect on BP, reinforcing reports that aldosterone excess may worsen obstructive sleep apnea by promoting the accumulation of fluid within the neck, which then contributes to increase upper airway resistance [17]. In addition, excessive dietary sodium intake contributes to the development of resistant hypertension both through directly increasing BP and by blunting the BP-lowering effect of most classes of antihypertensive agents [18]. Recently, Pimenta et al. [19] have shown that mean office systolic BP (SBP) and diastolic BP (DBP) were reduced by 22.7 and 9.1 mmHg, respectively, during low- compared with high-salt diets provided to resistant hypertensive patients. This indicates that excessive dietary sodium ingestion contributes substantially to resistance to antihypertensive treatment. The DASH diet reduced SBP and DBP by 11.4 and 5.5 mmHg, respectively, more than the control diet in hypertensive patients, but the benefit of this diet has not been evaluated separately in patients with resistant hypertension [5, 11]. Regular aerobic exercise, which may produce mean reductions of 4 mmHg in SBP and 3 mmHg in DBP [20], and cessation of heavy alcohol ingestion can significantly improve hypertension control. Therefore, all the strategies based on lifestyle changes should be part of the overall treatment for resistant hypertension. However, as their real implementation and effectiveness require behavioral support, counseling, and reinforcement, the costs may be substantial. As far as we know, no studies of the cost-effectiveness of non-pharmacological treatment have been reported so far in patients with resistant hypertension.

15.3 Cost-Effectiveness of Pharmacological Treatment in Resistant Hypertensive Patients

Treatment recommendations in patients with resistant hypertension cannot be overly standardized, particularly when going beyond 3 drugs. By definition, resistant hypertensive subjects must be taking optimal doses of at least 3 classes of antihypertensive drugs, including a diuretic [5, 11]. In most countries, a diuretic is the cheapest option to treat hypertension and is therefore the most cost-effective. Studies have demonstrated additive antihypertensive effects by combining two agents of different classes. This is particularly true for thiazide diuretics, which significantly improve BP control when used in combination with most, if not all, other classes of antihypertensive agents. In this respect, a triple-drug regimen including an angiotensin-converting enzyme inhibitor (ACEi) or/and angiotensin II receptor blocker (ARB), a calcium channel blocker, and a thiazide diuretic is very effective in reducing BP values and cardiovascular morbidity and mortality and is generally well tolerated [5, 11].

In addition, this combination of drugs has been shown to regress left ventricular hypertrophy, although a greater reduction in microalbuminuria or proteinuria has been found by blocking the renin–angiotensin system with ACEi or ARB [21–23]. In this respect, for equivalent BP lowering within each class of ACEI, ARB, and CCB, the least expensive is the most cost-effective drug.

Studies have shown that spironolactone lowers SBP and DBP by 24 and 10 mmHg, respectively, when added to the regimen of patients with BP uncontrolled with at least two medications [24, 25]. Likewise, mineralocorticoid receptor blockade induces rapid regression of left ventricular hypertrophy irrespective of aldosterone status [26]. Furthermore, there is increasing evidence linking aldosterone with both resistant hypertension and obstructive sleep apnea, with preliminary studies suggesting that aldosterone antagonists may potentially be effective in treating both conditions. Finally, especially in very high-risk patients who obtain large benefits from lowering BP, treatment with multiple drugs, even those that are expensive, might also be cost-effective [27]. As far as we know, no studies of the cost-effectiveness of pharmacological treatment have been reported so far in patients with resistant hypertension.

15.4 Cost-Effectiveness of the New Interventional Strategies in Resistant Hypertensive Patients

Recent studies have focused on novel invasive strategies for the management of resistant hypertension, specifically baroreflex activation therapy with carotid stimulation and percutaneous renal artery denervation (RDN). The use of these approaches has shown to be safe and effective in clinical trials. Catheter-based RDN has proven to be effective and safe in reducing BP in resistant hypertensive patients during at least two years [28, 29] and can also improve glucose metabolism and insulin sensitivity [30]. Likewise, baroreflex activation therapy has shown its efficacy and safety in resistant hypertensive subjects with multiple comorbidities, and with different therapies, in the long term [31, 32].

As stated, the increasing limitations on healthcare budgets and the rising costs of health care, particularly those caused by new therapeutic approaches, make an evaluation of cost-effectiveness advisable for every new technique [33]. Cost-benefit analysis of these new treatments should take some singularities into account. Costs should refer to the total expenditures related to treatment, as in classical management, but also to the cost of these techniques (renal denervation or baroreflex activation therapy) in themselves. This should include the costs for the device, surgical implantation or removal, and ongoing maintenance. Analysis of benefits should focus on future possible savings due to the prevention of disease morbidity and mortality and the reduction in the costs of hospitalization and care for diseases caused by resistant hypertension including end-stage renal disease, myocardial infarction, heart failure, stroke, intracerebral hemorrhage, subarachnoid hemorrhage, and transient ischemic attack.

As in all analyses of this type, the main limitation is the variability in costs and differences in practice that may vary considerably between regions or providers. This difficulty could be addressed in part by performing sensitivity analyses and ranges or by estimating average costs. However, it is not easy to measure effectiveness. While the relative weight of every disease on outcomes has to be taken in account, benefits should be measured in units that are relevant to these interventions. These units should reflect cardiovascular events prevented, lives saved, and life-years gained. Thus, the use of quality-adjusted life-years (QALYs) gained reflects the prolongation and quality of life associated with the years gained.

As it is a recently introduced technique, cost-benefit data on baroreflex activation therapy with carotid stimulation and percutaneous RDN are scarce.

Recently, Young et al. [34] reported the results of a study designed to investigate the cost-effectiveness of an implantable carotid body stimulator (Rheos; CVRx, Inc., Minneapolis, MN) in the treatment for resistant hypertension and to determine the range of starting SBP values where the device remains cost-effective. The authors used a Markov model incorporating future adverse events (event rates for future death, stroke, heart failure, end-stage renal disease, or myocardial infarction), costs, and benefits and compared a fall in SBP with the Rheos implantable device of up to 20 mmHg from different initial levels in patients who failed medical management. The analysis was performed in a hypothetical asymptomatic 50-year-old cohort with uncontrolled resistant hypertension and no history of CV disease or stroke. The authors found an incremental cost-effectiveness ratio (ICER) for the Rheos device of $64,400 per QALY. Analysis of different scenarios depending on baseline BP values (140–220 mmHg) showed that the ICER was <$100,000 per QALY for patients with the lowest initial SBP. Systolic BP reductions >24 mmHg reduced the ICER to > $50,000 per QALY. When a cohort with clinical characteristics similar to that of the Anglo-Scandinavian Cardiac Outcomes Trial-Blood Pressure Lowering Arm (ASCOT-BPLA), namely patients with hypertension and at least three additional cardiovascular risk factors but no history of coronary heart disease was used, the ICER was reduced to \$26,700 per QALY. The authors concluded that the Rheos device may be cost-effective, with an ICER between \$50,000 and \$100,000 per QALY.

Geisler et al. have very recently reported the results of a study designed to assess the cost-effectiveness and long-term clinical benefits of RDN in resistant hypertensive patients and identify the subgroups in which this therapy is clinically most efficacious and cost-effective [35]. They retrospectively analyzed data from the randomized controlled Symplicity HTN-2 trial which included 106 patients, with a mean age of 58 ± 12 years, of whom 34 % were diabetic and 16 % of smokers, and with a mean baseline SBP of 178 ± 17 mmHg. On average, catheter-based RDN lowered SBP by 32 ± 23 mmHg from baseline.

The study used covariates that were identified as statistically significant ($p < 0.05$) by a bi-/multivariate linear regression analysis to develop a predictive model. A state transition model was used to predict the effect of RDN plus the standard of care compared with standard of care only (pharmacological treatment) on 10-year and lifetime probabilities of stroke, myocardial infarction and coronary heart disease, heart failure, end-stage renal disease, and median survival (Fig. 15.1). The analyses were conducted using a lifetime horizon and the cost-effectiveness ratio (ICER) defined as the incremental direct medical costs of

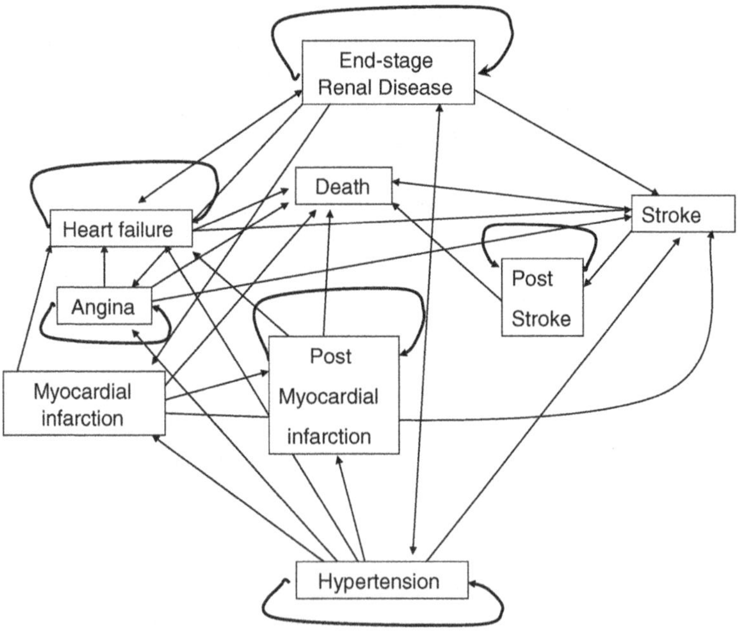

Fig. 15.1 Markov model for renal denervation cost-effectiveness analysis, with a simulated cohort of patients with resistant hypertension but no prior cardiovascular disease. Cohort members can reach more than one of stroke, myocardial infarction, angina, heart failure, end-stage renal disease, and death. Modified with permission from [35]

treatment and consequences in 2010 US dollars divided by the incremental health benefits expressed as quality-adjusted life-years (QALYs). Deterministic sensitivity analyses were used to quantify the effect of covariates on the ICER. Baseline SBP was used as a predictive covariate.

With respect to effectiveness in reducing events (Table 15.1), RDN substantially reduced event probabilities, with the following lifetime relative risks: stroke 0.83; heart failure 0.92; myocardial infarction 0.85; all coronary heart disease 0.90; end-stage renal disease 0.81. Median survival was 18.4 years for RDN versus 17.1 years for standard of care. The discounted lifetime ICER was $3,071 per QALY. The probabilistic sensitivity analysis indicated a 97 % chance of the ICER being <$30,000 per QALY in the cohort analyzed and a 99.6 % probability that the ICER being <$50,000 per QALY threshold. The model suggests that catheter-based RDN, over a wide range of assumptions, is a cost-effective strategy for resistant hypertension that might result in lower cardiovascular morbidity and mortality. The authors concluded that percutaneous RDN seemed not only to be clinically efficacious, but also to be cost-effective across a broad range of baseline SBP values.

Table 15.1 Prediction of reduction in the risk of clinical events in the base case for renal denervation versus standard of care and cost-effectiveness analysis. Modified with permission from [35]

Lifetime Horizon				
Base case	Standard of care (%)	Renal denervation (%)	Risk difference (%)	Relative risk
Cerebrovascular disease				
Stroke	31.9	26.4	5.5	0.83
Heart disease				
Heart failure	14.1	13.0	1.1	0.92
Myocardial infarction	31.0	26.2	4.7	0.85
Coronary heart disease	55.3	49.6	5.7	0.90
Renal disease				
End-stage renal disease	5.5	4.4	1.1	0.92
Median survival	17.07	18.37	1.30	1.08
QALYs	12.07	13.17	1.10	1.09
Discounted ICER		3071 US$/QALY		

ICER incremental cost-effectiveness ratio
QALYs quality-adjusted life-years

In summary, RDN seems to be more cost-effective (ICER between $30,000 and $50,000 per QALY) than carotid baroreceptor stimulation (ICER between $50,000 and $100,000 per QALY) in patients with resistant hypertension. Although RDN therapy represents an additional cost at the time of treatment, it seems to offer great value over time.

References

1. Dahlöf B, Hansson L, Lindholm L, Råstam L, Scherstén B, Wester PO (1986) STOP-hypertension: swedish trial in old patients with hypertension. J Hypertens 4:511–513
2. SHEP Cooperative Research Group (1991) Prevention of stroke by antihypertensive drug treatment in older persons with isolated systolic hypertension. Final results of the systolic hypertension in the elderly program (SHEP). JAMA 265:3255–3264
3. Amery A, Birkenhäger W, Bogaert M, Brixko P, Bulpitt C, Clement D, De Leeuw P, De Plaen JF, Deruyttere M, De Schaepdryver A, Fagard R, Forette F, Forte J, Hamdy R, Hellemans J, Henry JF, Koistinen A, Laaser U, Laher M, Leonetti G, Lewis P, Lund-Johansen P, MacFarlane J, Meurer K, Miguel P, Morris J, Mutsers A, Nissinen A, O'Brien E, Ohm OJ, O'Malley K, Pelemans W, Perera N, Tuomilehto J, Verschueren LJ, Willemse P, Williams B, Zanchetti A (1982) Antihypertensive therapy in patients above age 60 with systolic hypertension. A progress report of the European working party on high blood pressure in the elderly (EWPHE). Clin Exp Hypertens 4:1151–1176
4. Sytkowski PA, D'Agostino RB, Belanger AJ, Kannel WB (1996) Secular trends in long-term sustained hypertension, long-term treatment, and cardiovascular mortality. The Framingham Heart Study 1950 to 1990. Circulation 1996(93):697–703
5. Mancia G, De Backer G, Dominiczak A, Cifkova R, Fagard R, Germano G et al (2007) 2007 ESH-ESC practice guidelines for the management of arterial hypertension: ESH-ESC Task force on the management of arterial hypertension. J Hypertens 25:1751–1762
6. Hedner T (1998) Treating hypertension–effect of treatment and cost-effectiveness in respect to later cardiovascular diseases. Scand Cardiovasc J 47(Supplement):31–35
7. Law MR, Morris JK, Wald NJ (2009) Use of blood pressure lowering drugs in the prevention of cardiovascular disease: meta-analysis of 147 randomised trials in the context of expectations from prospective epidemiological studies. BMJ 338:b1665–b1683
8. Dickinson HO, Mason JM, Nicolson DJ, Campbell F, Beyer FR, Cook JV et al (2006) Lifestyle interventions to reduce raised blood pressure: a systematic review of randomized controlled trials. J Hypertens 24:215–233
9. National Kidney Foundation (2004) Executive summary. Am J Kid Dis 43(Suppl. 1):S16–S33
10. Mann JF, Gerstein HC, Pogue J, Bosch J, Yusuf S (2001) Renal insufficiency as a predictor of cardiovascular outcomes and the impact of ramipril: the HOPE randomized trial. Ann Intern Med 134:629–636
11. Calhoun DA, Jones D, Textor S, Goff DC, Murphy TP, Toto RD et al (2008) Resistant hypertension: diagnosis, evaluation, and treatment. A scientific statement from the American heart association professional education committee of the council for high blood pressure research. Hypertension 51:1403–1419
12. Salles GF, Cardoso CR, Muxfeldt ES (2008) Prognostic influence of office and ambulatory blood pressures in resistant hypertension. Arch Intern Med 168:2340–2346
13. Cushman WC, Ford CE, Cutler JA, Margolis KL, Davis BR, Grimm RH et al (2002) Success and predictors of blood pressure control in diverse North American settings: the antihypertensive and lipid-lowering treatment to prevent heart attack trial (ALLHAT). J Clin Hypertens (Greenwich). 4:393–404

14. Bramlage P, Pittrow D, Wittchen HU, Kirch W, Boehler S, Lehnert H et al (2004) Hypertension in overweight and obese primary care patients is highly prevalent and poorly controlled. Am J Hypertens 17:904–910
15. Nishizaka MK, Pratt-Ubunama M, Zaman MA, Cofield S, Calhoun DA (2005) Validity of plasma aldosterone-to-renin activity ratio in African American and white subjects with resistant hypertension. Am J Hypertens 18:805–812
16. Pedrosa RP, Drager LF, Gonzaga CC, Sousa MG, de Paula LK, Amaro AC et al (2011) Obstructive sleep apnea: the most common secondary cause of hypertension associated with resistant hypertension. Hypertension 58:811–817
17. Dudenbostel T, Calhoun DA (2012) Resistant hypertension, obstructive sleep apnoea and aldosterone. J Hum Hypertens 26:281–287
18. Weinberger MH, Cohen SJ, Miller JZ, Luft FC, Grim CE, Fineberg NS (1988) Dietary sodium restriction as adjunctive treatment of hypertension. JAMA 259:2561–2565
19. Pimenta E, Gaddam KK, Oparil S, Aban I, Husain S, Dell'Italia LJ et al (2009) Effects of dietary sodium reduction on blood pressure in subjects with resistant hypertension: results from a randomized trial. Hypertension 54:475–481
20. Whelton SP, Chin A, Xin X, He J (2002) Effect of aerobic exercise on blood pressure: a meta-analysis of randomized, controlled trials. Ann Intern Med 136:493–503
21. Dahlöf B, Devereux RB, Kjeldsen SE, Julius S, Beevers G, de Faire U et al (2002) Cardiovascular morbidity and mortality in the Losartan intervention for endpoint reduction in hypertension study (LIFE): a randomised trial against atenolol. Lancet 359:995–1003
22. Schmieder RE, Schlaich MP, Klingbeil AU, Martus P (1998) Update on reversal of left ventricular hypertrophy in essential hypertension (a meta-analysis of all randomized double-blind studies until December 1996). Nephrol Dial Transplant 13:564–569
23. Devereux RB, Palmieri V, Sharpe N, De Quattro V, Bella JN, de Simone G et al (2001) Effects of once-daily angiotensin-converting enzyme inhibition and calcium channel blockade-based antihypertensive treatment regimens on left ventricular hypertrophy and diastolic filling in hypertension: the prospective randomized enalapril study evaluating regression of ventricular enlargement (preserve) trial. Circulation 104:1248–1254
24. Ouzan J, Pérault C, Lincoff AM, Carré E, Mertes M (2002) The role of spironolactone in the treatment of patients with refractory hypertension. Am J Hypertens 15:333–339
25. Ubaid-Girioli S, Adriana de Souza L, Yugar-Toledo JC, Martins LC, Ferreira-Melo S, Coelho OR, Sierra C, Coca A, Pimenta E, Moreno H (2009) Aldosterone excess or escape: treating resistant hypertension. J Clin Hypertens (Greenwich) 11:245–252
26. Gaddam K, Corros C, Pimenta E, Ahmed M, Denney T, Aban I, Inusah S, Gupta H, Lloyd SG, Oparil S, Husain A, Dell'Italia LJ, Calhoun DA (2010) Rapid reversal of left ventricular hypertrophy and intracardiac volume overload in patients with resistant hypertension and hyperaldosteronism: a prospective clinical study. Hypertension 55:1137–1142
27. Lindholm L, Hallgren CG, Boman K, Markgren K, Weinehall L, Ogren JE (1999) Cost-effectiveness analysis with defined budget: how to distribute resources for the prevention of cardiovascular disease? Health Policy 48:155–170
28. Esler MD, Krum H, Sobotka PA, Schlaich MP, Schmieder RE, Böhm M et al (2010) Renal sympathetic denervation in patients with treatment-resistant hypertension (The Simplicity HTN-2 Trial): a randomised controlled trial. Lancet 376:1903–1909
29. Symplicity HTN-1 Investigators (2011) Catheter-based renal sympathetic denervation for resistant hypertension: durability of blood pressure reduction out to 24 months. Hypertension 57:911–917
30. Mahfoud F, Schlaich M, Kindermann I, Ukena C, Cremers B, Brandt MC et al (2011) Effect of renal sympathetic denervation on glucose metabolism in patients with resistant hypertension: a pilot study. Circulation 123:1940–1946
31. Scheffers IJ, Kroon AA, Schmidli J, Jordan J, Tordoir JJ, Mohaupt MG et al (2010) Baroreflex activation therapy in resistant hypertension: results of a European multi-center feasibility study. J Am Coll Cardiol 56:1254–1258

32. Bisognano JD, Bakris G, Nadim MK, Sanchez L, Kroon AA, Schafer J et al (2011) Baroreflex activation therapy lowers blood pressure in patients with resistant hypertension: results from the double-blind, randomized, placebo-controlled RHEOS pivotal trial. J Am Coll Cardiol 58:765–773
33. American College of Physicians (2008) Information on cost-effectiveness: an essential product of a national comparative effectiveness program. Ann Intern Med 148:956–961
34. Young KC, Teeters JC, Benesch CG, Bisognano JD, Illig KA (2009) Cost-effectiveness of treating resistant hypertension with an implantable carotid body stimulator. J Clin Hypertens (Greenwich) 11:555–563
35. Geisler BP, Egan BM, Cohen JT, Garner AM, Akehurst RL, Esler MD et al (2012) Cost-effectiveness and clinical effectiveness of catheter-based renal denervation for resistant hypertension. J Am Coll Cardiol Article in press. doi: 10.1016/j.jacc.2012.07.029

16 Involvement of Health Professionals: From the General Practitioner to the Hypertension Specialist and the Hypertension Center

Massimo Volpe and Giuliano Tocci

16.1 Introduction

Resistant hypertension is a very complex disease [1]. Its pathophysiology is characterized by persistently high blood pressure (BP) levels above the recommended BP goals (i.e., below 140/90 mmHg) in the presence of lifestyle changes and optimal antihypertensive strategy based on at least three antihypertensive agents, including a diuretic at adequate doses [2]. It is often associated with the presence of organ damage, including left ventricular hypertrophy and/or dysfunction, carotid or peripheral atherosclerosis, albuminuria or renal impairment, and leads to higher susceptibility to develop overt cardiovascular and renal complications, including myocardial infarction, stroke, congestive heart failure, and end-stage renal disease [2]. As such, this condition is associated with higher risk of cardiovascular morbidity and mortality than essential hypertension and deserves specific pharmacological and non-pharmacological interventions to reduce this risk.

Conflict of Interest Statement: MV has received research grants from Novartis, has served in international advisory boards of Daiichi Sankyo, Menarini, Malesci, Guidotti, and Novartis Farma, and has lectured in symposia supported by several drug companies producing ARBs and ACE Inhibitors; GT has no conflict of interest to disclose. MV is a member of a Medtronic Global Simplicity Registry; GT has no conflict of interest to disclose.

M. Volpe (✉) · G. Tocci
Department of Clinical and Molecular Medicine, University of Rome "Sapienza", Sant'Andrea Hospital, Via di Grottarossa 1035-9, 00189 Rome, Italy
e-mail: massimo.volpe@uniroma1.it

G. Tocci
e-mail: giuliano.tocci@uniroma1.it

G. Mancia (ed.), *Resistant Hypertension*, DOI: 10.1007/978-88-470-5415-8_16,

Achieving effective and sustained BP control is obviously paralleled by a marked reduction in fatal and non-fatal outcomes in these patients, as well as in those with essential hypertension [3–5]. However, in patients with resistant hypertension, it is more difficult to reduce BP levels to targets than in patients with essential hypertension, even in the presence of more complex and integrated antihypertensive strategies, including four to five antihypertensive agents of different classes.

Several reasons can be advocated to explain why BP remains persistently high, and several pharmacological [6–9] and non-pharmacological [11, 12] options have been proposed and tested to reduce systolic and diastolic BP levels in these patients with challenging or difficult-to-treat hypertension. A difficult control of BP levels in patients with resistant hypertension may, indeed, be related to factors including doctors' inertia, patients' poor adherence to prescribed pharmacological therapy, insufficient patient–doctor communication, inappropriate BP measurements, or inadequate or insufficient antihypertensive interventions [13].

Whatever the case, it is quite evident that these patients need a multidisciplinary and integrated clinical approach to ensure persistence on favorable lifestyle measures, high adherence to prescribed antihypertensive therapy and accurate out-of-office (home and ambulatory) BP measurements.

In this chapter, we will discuss the potential impact of a multidisciplinary and multidimensional approach for improving BP control in patients with resistant or refractory hypertension and the role of different professional figures involved in the clinical management of hypertension in this high-risk population. We will also briefly address the importance of counseling from trained nurses and the key role of patients' relatives among non-pharmacologic interventions, which may help to achieve better BP control and improve adherence to prescribed therapy in patients with resistant forms of hypertension. Although of clinical relevance, particularly in view of the progressively high incidence of this clinical condition in the general population of hypertensive patients, these aspects have never been addressed in the medical literature and marginally discussed in international current guidelines for hypertension diagnosis and treatment [2, 14, 15].

16.2 Modern and Integrated Approach to Treat Patients with Resistant Hypertension

A modern approach for the clinical management of patients with resistant or refractory hypertension should include not only the implementation of lifestyle change, the use of pharmacological (rational, synergistic, and effective combination therapies) and non-pharmacological (renal artery denervation or carotid baroreflex stimulation) interventions, but also the interactions among different professional figures. These multiple and reciprocal interactions among different professional figures share several common aims, including: (1) reducing BP levels to targets, if tolerated and not contraindicated; (2) limiting the progression of hypertension-related organ damage; (3) preserving cardiac and renal function in individual patients with resistant hypertension.

It should be highlighted, however, that resistant hypertension is not a "numbers' disease," and limiting therapeutic actions to merely lowering absolute BP levels may not correspond to a clinical success. In other words, physicians should not focus their attention only on the markedly high BP levels and on the effort of achieving the most effective and rapid BP reductions. Yet, they should aim at reducing individual global cardiovascular risk profile, mostly by lowering BP levels, as recommended by current guidelines [2].

In this latter regard, European guidelines proposed a new clinical approach and targets for the clinical management of cardiovascular risk factors, including hypertension [2, 16], moving from the so-called silos approach to an "integrated" approach, aimed at reducing individual global cardiovascular risk rather than absolute levels of individual risk factors in isolation, in this case high BP levels [17]. A similar integrated approach should be also proposed even for the involvement of different professional figures in the clinical management of patients with resistant hypertension.

Even in this clinical setting, in fact, physicians' interventions in the individual patient should move beyond the traditional approach aimed at lowering absolute BP levels by individually adding the prescriptions from "cardiologists," "nephrologists," "endocrinologists," or "general practitioners" in the so-called silos approach, toward a new, integrated, and multidisciplinary approach that may lead to get a more thorough estimation of cardiovascular risk, which is currently defined as "total" or "global" cardiovascular risk [17]. Accordingly, physicians with different professional figures and skills should simultaneously act on a number of different pathophysiological factors involved in the development and progression of resistant hypertension, sharing pharmacological and non-pharmacological therapies for achieving effective and sustained BP reductions. A tentative list of professional, both medical and paramedical, figures that may be involved in the clinical management of resistant hypertension is reported on Table 16.1. This will translate into a new therapeutic approach, not only based on the synergistic and effective involvement of different professional figures separately, but rather based on a multidisciplinary and multidimensional approach, which involved different professional figures under the supervision of certified hypertension specialists, as schematically represented in Fig. 16.1.

16.2.1 Hypertension Specialist

Hypertension specialist should have a leading role in the clinical management of patients with resistant hypertension, in view of her/his certified expertise in treating patients with severe hypertension, marked degree of organ damage, and associated clinical conditions. Current European guidelines, in fact, recommended that patients who do not respond to standard antihypertensive regimen, which

Table 16.1 Professional (medical and paramedical) figures that should be involved in the clinical management of resistant hypertension.

Medical figures	Paramedical figures
• Hypertension specialists	• Trained Nurses
• Cardiologists	• Sonographers
• Nephrologists	• Dietitians
• Internists	• Pharmacists
• Geriatricians	• Paramedics who are specialized in Neuropathophysiology for nocturnal Polysomnography
• Endocrinologists (diabetologist)	
• Diagnostic and/or interventional radiologists	• Paramedics who are specialized in renal perfusion for hemodialysis
• Clinical biologists	
• Molecular biologists	
• Pneumologists	
• Psychologists	
• General practitioners	

Among these, hypertension specialist should have a central role in coordinating both pharmacological and non-pharmacological interventions to achieve effective and sustained blood pressure reductions

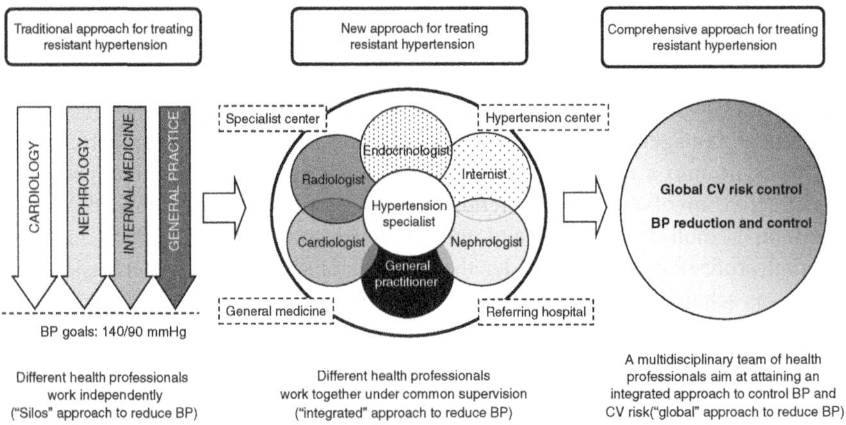

Fig. 16.1 Schematic representation of different professional figures involved in the clinical management of resistant hypertension. Traditional approach is characterized by individual interventions ("silos" approach) aimed at lowering blood pressure levels. New approach should be characterized by integrated and multidisciplinary interventions ("integrated" approach) for treating individual patients with resistant hypertension. Modified with permission from [17]

often includes one diuretic and at least one or two additional antihypertensive drug classes, independently by the class or the dosage, should be referred from general practitioners to hypertension excellence centers [2].

At this level, patients with difficult-to-treat or challenging hypertension can be re-evaluated by hypertension specialists for global cardiovascular risk profile assessment, exclusion of pseudo-resistance hypertension, search for secondary causes of hypertension, and implementation or optimization of combination therapies. Being the majority of these patients within the diagnostic criteria of resistant or refractory hypertension [2], hypertension specialist may play a central role in: (1) confirming the diagnosis of true resistance to pharmacological treatment through accurate clinic and out-of-office (home and ambulatory) BP monitoring; (2) excluding secondary causes of hypertension by advanced diagnostic examinations; (3) verifying patent's adherence to prescribed antihypertensive therapy, and (4) implementing effective, safe, and well-tolerated therapeutic strategies, mostly including rational and synergistic combination therapies and non-pharmacological interventions, if appropriate.

First of all, it is of key relevance that hypertension specialist must systematically exclude the presence of the so-called pseudo-resistance hypertension, which can be often undiagnosed with first-line examinations. Several factors can be advocated for explaining the "pseudo-resistance" hypertension, among which heavily calcified or arteriosclerotic arteries in elderly subjects, "white-coat" effect, poor patient adherence to prescribed therapy, side effects or adverse reactions of medications, complex dosing schedules, poor communication between doctor and patient, inadequate patient education, memory or psychiatric problems, costs of medication, inadequate doses or inappropriate combination therapies, physician inertia (failure to change or increase dose regimens when not at goal). Proper clinic BP measurements, associated with 24-h ambulatory BP monitoring, performed according to current guidelines' recommendations [18], can be useful for identifying potential causes of pseudo-resistance hypertension. All these factors should be obviously removed to confirm the diagnosis of true resistant hypertension.

The availability of advanced diagnostic tools (e.g., tissue Doppler imaging, 3D-echocardiogram, high-sensitivity peripheral Doppler ultrasound examination, angio-cardiac tomography and magnetic resonance) as well as hematological, immunohistochemical, and neurohormonal assays (dosage of neurohormones, including adrenaline, noradrenaline, renin, aldosterone, plasma renin-activity, and natriuretic peptides) may also help for more accurate, although more expensive, diagnostic evaluation of patients with resistant or refractory hypertension and for excluding secondary causes of hypertension (e.g., hyperaldosteronism).

It should be also noted, however, that it may not be cost-effective and that it may be not rational to prescribe all these advanced diagnostic examinations to each patient with a clinical suspicion of treatment resistance. In this view, hypertension specialist should select proper diagnostic and clinical examinations according to the individual global cardiovascular risk profile and clinical judgment.

In view of the pathophysiological complexity and the heterogeneity of clinical presentation of resistant hypertension, the clinical management of this condition should be implemented by other professional figures and consultants, who may provide specialized support during the decision-making process and diagnostic and therapeutic algorhythms.

16.2.2 Specialized Physicians

The pathogenesis of resistant hypertension is extremely complex and often related to concomitant interactions of different pathophysiological mechanisms that may contribute to maintain high BP levels, despite optimal antihypertensive therapy. In addition, clinical signs or symptoms may substantially vary, depending of the involvement of different organs or apparatus. In view of this pathophysiological complexity and clinical heterogeneity, several other professional figures are often involved in the clinical management of this high-risk clinical condition, besides the central role of hypertension specialists.

First of all, cardiologists are primarily involved in the clinical management of patients with resistant hypertension in view of the frequent concomitant presence of cardiac organ damage, including left ventricular hypertrophy or dysfunction [19]. In this clinical setting, the contribution of cardiologist should be of particular relevance for: (1) careful assessment of cardiac function throughout functional and provocative tests (i.e., echocardiography, eco-stress imaging, provocative or stress test with treadmill, or cycloergometer); (2) proper recommendations for daily physical exercise, according to functional status of the heart; (3) titration of the appropriate dose of antihypertensive therapy. In particular, the use of full dose of either Angiotensin-Converting Enzyme (ACE) inhibitors or Angiotensin Receptor Blockers (ARBs) is often required in patients with resistant hypertension and evidence of left ventricular hypertrophy or dysfunction, in order to promote regression or limiting the progression of cardiac organ damage [20]. Also, cardiologists should work to exclude the concomitant presence of coronary artery disease, since this may have potential clinical implications for the clinical management of patients with resistant hypertension [21]. Evidence of myocardial ischemia due to coronary atherosclerosis may, in fact, represent a major contraindication for aggressive and extreme BP reductions (i.e., BP below 130/80 mmHg), because there are conflicting evidence for extreme lowering BP levels in this clinical setting [21].

Nephrologists are often involved in the clinical management of patients with resistant hypertension, in view of the frequent concomitant presence of renal damage, as defined by the presence of microalbuminuria, proteinuria, or reduced glomerular filtration rate [2]. In this clinical setting, the contribution of nephrologist should be of particular relevance for: (1) careful assessment of renal function throughout functional and diagnostic examinations; (2) proper recommendations for daily sodium and water assumption by diet, according to 24-h urine analysis;

(3) titration of the appropriate dose of diuretic therapy. In this latter regard, since patients with resistant hypertension require the use of at least one class of diuretic, independently by the class or the dosage, this may lead to underuse or under dosage of combination of two (or three) classes of diuretics (i.e., thiazide or loop diuretics, antialdosterone agents). It should be also noted that in the daily clinical practice, it is quite common the use of "inadequate" doses of diuretic drugs (for example, hydrochlorothiazide 12.5 mg/once daily), or the use of a thiazide-like diuretic with a longer half-life (e.g., chlorthalidone 25 mg/once daily), administered either as a stand-alone drug (monotherapy) or as a combination drug (combination therapy). Such doses or strategies are inadequate to achieve and maintain effective BP control over time, mostly in patients with a glomerular filtration rate below 30 ml/min and in those categories of hypertensive patients with a high cardiovascular risk, such as elderly or diabetic patients. The correct titration of the diuretics to "adequate" doses (e.g., hydrochlorothiazide 25 mg/ once daily) is an essential step to improve BP control and to properly identify patients with true resistant hypertension. Nephrologists can be also involved for up-titrating the dosage of renin–angiotensin system blocking agents, including Angiotensin-Converting Enzyme (ACE) inhibitors and Angiotensin Receptor Blockers (ARBs), which have demonstrated to promote regression of proteinuria or even normalization of normal buminuria, when used at full dose [22–24]. Finally, nephrologists may be asked to contribute to rule out the diagnosis of secondary hypertension or renal origin.

Internists or geriatricians are also involved in the clinical management of patients with resistant hypertension. In view of the progressive aging of the global general population, particularly in Western Countries and in view of the frequent presence of concomitant cardiovascular and non-cardiovascular diseases, as well as of the frequent use of concomitant cardiovascular and non-cardiovascular drugs (e.g., aspirin, lipid-lowering drugs, hormone replacement therapy, non-steroidal anti-inflammatory agents, corticosteroids, neuroleptic, and antipsychotic agents), a comprehensive and "internistic" approach to the hypertension-related problem should help in identifying potential secondary (drug-induced) causes of resistant hypertension. In this clinical setting, the contribution of internists or geriatricians should be of particular relevance for: (1) careful assessment of central or peripheral vascular function throughout imaging tests (i.e., carotid or femoral vascular Doppler ultrasound, pulse wave velocity, central aortic pressure, pletismography); (2) proper recommendations for daily physical activity, according to functional and neurological status; (3) identification of potential unfavorable or negative interactions among drugs and prescriptions of rational combination therapies.

Endocrinologists play a key role in the identification or rule out of relatively common forms of secondary hypertension, such as hyperaldosteronism CR10, whereas diabetologists are today frequently asked to be part of the team of physicians approaching patients with resistant hypertension, due to the frequent concomitance in the same subject of glucose metabolism disorders and type 2 diabetes, as well as for the work-up and follow-up designed to prevent the complications of the deleterious correlation between hypertension and diabetes.

16.2.3 General Practitioner

Although guidelines state that the clinical management of patients with resistant hypertension should be referred to hypertension specialists who have practice in hypertension excellence centers, the role of general practitioners and the contribution of general medicine is of key relevance and cannot be discussed. An active and effective collaboration between hypertension center and referring general practitioner may provide a reciprocal and favorable link, in order to: (1) improve patients' adherence to prescribed antihypertensive strategy; (2) avoid inappropriate and expensive hospital admission for "hypertensive crisis," which often does not require any other intervention than prescription of oral antihypertensive therapy; (3) ensure proper BP measurements, according to current guidelines' recommendations [25].

16.2.4 Trained Nurses

The clinical management of patients with resistant or refractory hypertension should not avoid the fundamental contribution of nurses, who are trained for different techniques of BP measurements. Appropriate clinic BP measurement, in fact, is a fundamental step for confirming the diagnosis of true resistant hypertension. In view of the well-known influence of physicians' presence ("white-coat effect") [26], as well as of other confounding factors (e.g., anxiety, noises, tremors), improper or inaccurate BP measurements should be always considered as potential causes of pseudo-resistance hypertension.

In addition, since patients with true resistant hypertension often require repeated 24-h ambulatory BP monitoring, counseling of trained nurses may ensure high-quality BP recordings over the entire 24 h. This is of particular relevance to evaluate 24-h BP control of a given antihypertensive strategy, particularly during the nighttime period and awake, during which the risk of developing major cardiovascular events, mostly stroke, is higher than the rest of the day [27].

Finally, trained nurses may have a fundamental role for accurate and systematic home BP monitoring [28]. This should be obtained by properly counseling of patients with resistant hypertension, who obviously need a careful assessment of BP profile at home, in order to verify effective and sustained BP control over time.

16.2.5 Other Professional Figures and the Role of Relatives

Several other professional, paramedical figures can be involved in the clinical management of patients with resistant or refractory hypertension (Table 16.1). For example, it has been reported a higher prevalence of obstructive sleep apnea syndrome in patients with true resistant hypertension compared to patients with essential hypertension [29]. As a consequence, patients with resistant hypertension often require nocturnal polysomnography or pulsoximetry to evaluate apnea-hypopnoea index and the eventual indication of mechanical support for ventilation, such as continuous positive air pressure (cPAP). It has been also reported a higher prevalence of end-stage renal disease (ESRD) and dialysis in patients with resistant hypertension compared to those with essential hypertension. Thus, having information on water and sodium delivery during dialytic process may have provided useful information for proper titration of concomitant antihypertensive strategies, particularly for diuretic therapy. Finally, it has been recently emerged the relevant role of pharmacists for "out-of-office" BP measurements, which may represent a valid help for verifying the antihypertensive efficacy over the 24 h and improving patients' adherence to prescribed therapy.

16.3 Conclusions

Worldwide prevalence of hypertension is elevated, and BP control in hypertensive population remains unacceptably poor. This has dramatic consequences for public health, because the benefit of antihypertensive treatment is mostly related to the degree of systolic or diastolic BP reduction. The situation is even more dramatic in perspective, because of the continuing rise in the prevalence of hypertension and other comorbidities at global level.

The lack of BP control may be related to several factors, including doctors' inertia, patients' poor compliance, insufficient patient–doctor communication, inappropriate measurements of blood pressure, or inadequate or insufficient antihypertensive interventions.

Several reasons can be advocated to explain why BP remains persistently high and several pharmacological and non-pharmacological options have been proposed and tested to reduce systolic and diastolic BP levels in these patients with challenging or difficult-to-treat hypertension. Whatever the case, it is quite evident that these patients need a multidisciplinary and integrated approach to ensure persistence on favorable lifestyle measures, high adherence to prescribed antihypertensive therapy, and accurate out-of-office (home and ambulatory) BP measurements.

This multidisciplinary and multidimensional approach should help for improving BP control in patients with resistant or refractory hypertension throughout the reciprocal interactions among different professional figures, under the supervision of hypertension specialists involved in the clinical management of hypertension in this high-risk population.

References

1. Staessen JA, Wang J, Bianchi G, Birkenhager WH (2003) Essential hypertension. Lancet 361(9369):1629–1641
2. Mancia G, De Backer G, Dominiczak A, Cifkova R, Fagard R, Germano G et al (2007) ESH–ESC Practice guidelines for the management of arterial hypertension: ESH-ESC task force on the management of arterial hypertension. J Hypertens 25(9):1751–1762
3. Turnbull F, Neal B, Ninomiya T, Algert C, Arima H, Barzi F et al (2008) Effects of different regimens to lower blood pressure on major cardiovascular events in older and younger adults: meta-analysis of randomised trials. BMJ 336(7653):1121–1123
4. Turnbull F, Neal B, Algert C, Chalmers J, Chapman N, Cutler J et al (2005) Effects of different blood pressure-lowering regimens on major cardiovascular events in individuals with and without diabetes mellitus: results of prospectively designed overviews of randomized trials. Arch Intern Med 165(12):1410–1419
5. Turnbull F (2003) Effects of different blood-pressure-lowering regimens on major cardiovascular events: results of prospectively-designed overviews of randomised trials. Lancet 362(9395):1527–1535
6. de Souza F, Muxfeldt E, Fiszman R, Salles G (2010) Efficacy of spironolactone therapy in patients with true resistant hypertension. Hypertension 55(1):147–152
7. Rodilla E, Costa JA, Perez-Lahiguera F, Baldo E, Gonzalez C, Pascual JM (2009) Spironolactone and doxazosin treatment in patients with resistant hypertension. Rev Esp Cardiol 62(2):158–166
8. Oparil S, Melino M, Lee J, Fernandez V, Heyrman R (2010) Triple therapy with olmesartan medoxomil, amlodipine besylate, and hydrochlorothiazide in adult patients with hypertension: The TRINITY multicenter, randomized, double-blind, 12-week, parallel-group study. Clin Ther 32(7):1252–1269
9. Murray AV, Koenig W, Garcia-Puig J, Patel S, Phd AU, Zhang J (2012) Safety and efficacy of aliskiren/amlodipine/hydrochlorothiazide triple combination in patients with moderate to severe hypertension: a 54-week, open-label study. J Clin Hypertens (Greenwich) 14(12):821–827
10. Kittisupamongkol W (2009) Secondary causes of resistant hypertension. Arch Intern Med 169(7):717
11. Krum H, Schlaich M, Whitbourn R, Sobotka PA, Sadowski J, Bartus K et al (2009) Catheter-based renal sympathetic denervation for resistant hypertension: a multicentre safety and proof-of-principle cohort study. Lancet 373(9671):1275–1281
12. Mancia G, Parati G, Zanchetti A (2010) Electrical carotid baroreceptor stimulation in resistant hypertension. Hypertension
13. Volpe M, Tocci G (2010) Challenging hypertension: how to diagnose and treat resistant hypertension in daily clinical practice. Expert Rev Cardiovascular Ther 8(6):811–820
14. Chobanian AV, Bakris GL, Black HR, Cushman WC, Green LA, Izzo JL Jr et al (2003) The seventh report of the joint national committee on prevention, detection, evaluation, and treatment of high blood pressure: the JNC 7 report. JAMA 289(19):2560–2572
15. Williams B, Poulter NR, Brown MJ, Davis M, McInnes GT, Potter JF et al (2004) British hypertension society guidelines for hypertension management 2004 (BHS-IV): summary. BMJ 328(7440):634–640
16. Mancia G, Laurent S, Agabiti-Rosei E, Ambrosioni E, Burnier M, Caulfield MJ et al (2009) Reappraisal of European guidelines on hypertension management: a European society of hypertension task force document. J Hypertens 27(11):2121–2158
17. Volpe M, Erhardt LR, Williams B (2008) Managing cardiovascular risk: the need for change. J Hum Hypertens 22(2):154–157
18. O'Brien E, Asmar R, Beilin L, Imai Y, Mallion JM, Mancia G et al (2003) European society of hypertension recommendations for conventional, ambulatory and home blood pressure measurement. J Hypertens 21(5):821–848

19. Cuspidi C, Vaccarella A, Negri F, Sala C (2010) Resistant hypertension and left ventricular hypertrophy: an overview. J Am Soc Hypertens: JASH 4(6):319–324
20. Klingbeil AU, Schneider M, Martus P, Messerli FH, Schmieder RE (2003) A mcta-analysis of the effects of treatment on left ventricular mass in essential hypertension. Am J Med 115(1):41–46
21. Volpe M, Tocci G (2010) Rethinking targets of blood pressure and guidelines for hypertension clinical management. Nephrol Dial Transplant 25(11):3465–3471
22. Hollenberg NK, Parving HH, Viberti G, Remuzzi G, Ritter S, Zelenkofske S et al (2007) Albuminuria response to very high-dose valsartan in type 2 diabetes mellitus. J Hypertens 25(9):1921–1926
23. Makino H, Haneda M, Babazono T, Moriya T, Ito S, Iwamoto Y et al (2007) Prevention of transition from incipient to overt nephropathy with telmisartan in patients with type 2 diabetes. Diabetes Care 30(6):1577–1578
24. Ohishi M, Takagi T, Ito N, Tatara Y, Hayashi N, Shiota A et al (2007) Renal protective effect in hypertensive patients: the high doses of angiotensin II receptor blocker (HARB) study. Hypertens Res 30(12):1187–1192
25. O'Brien E, Asmar R, Beilin L, Imai Y, Mancia G, Mengden T et al (2005) Practice guidelines of the European society of hypertension for clinic, ambulatory and self blood pressure measurement. J Hypertens 23(4):697–701
26. Mancia G, Zanchetti A (1996) White-coat hypertension: misnomers, misconceptions and misunderstandings. What should we do next? J Hypertens 14(9):1049–1052
27. Elliott WJ (1998) Circadian variation in the timing of stroke onset: a meta-analysis. Stroke 29(5):992–996
28. Pickering TG, White WB, Giles TD, Black HR, Izzo JL, Materson BJ, et al (2010) When and how to use self (home) and ambulatory blood pressure monitoring. J Am Soc Hypertens: JASH 4(2):56–61
29. Pimenta E, Calhoun DA, Oparil S (2009) Sleep apnea, aldosterone, and resistant hypertension. Prog Cardiovasc Dis 51(5):371–380

Index

G. Mancia (ed.), *Resistant Hypertension*, DOI: 10.1007/978-88-470-5415-8,